T0317619

ICU CHEST RADIOLOGY

ICU CHEST RADIOLOGY
Principles and Case Studies

HAROLD MOSKOWITZ
University of Connecticut Health Center
Farmington, Connecticut

ⓦWILEY-BLACKWELL

A JOHN WILEY & SONS, INC., PUBLICATION

Wiley-Blackwell is an imprint of John Wiley & Sons, formed by the merger of Wiley's global Scientific, Technical, and Medical business with Blackwell Publishing.

Published by John Wiley & Sons, Inc., Hoboken, New Jersey
Published simultaneously in Canada

For general information on our other products and services or for technical support, please contact our Customer Care Department within the United States at (800) 762-2974, outside the United States at (317) 572-3993 or fax (317) 572-4002.

Wiley also publishes its books in a variety of electronic formats. Some content that appears in print may not be available in electronic formats. For more information about Wiley products, visit our web site at www.wiley.com.

Library of Congress Cataloging-in-Publication Data

Moskowitz, Harold.
    I.C.U. chest radiology : principles and case studies / Harold Moskowitz.
        p. ; cm.
    ISBN 978-0-470-45034-5 (cloth)
    1. Chest–Radiography–Case studies.   2. Chest–Diseases–Diagnosis–Case
studies.   3. Critical care medicine–Case studies.   I. Title.
    [DNLM: 1. Intensive Care Units–Case Reports.   2. Radiography, Thoracic–methods–
Case Reports.   3. Thoracic Diseases–diagnosis–Case Reports.   WX 218 M911i 2010]
    RC941.M67 2010
    617.5'407572–dc22
                                                                    2010001874

Printed in the United States of America

10 9 8 7 6 5 4 3 2 1

CONTENTS

*All of these case studies and the associated images are also located on the CD packaged with this book.

FOREWORD

Disclosure: The following story is true. And the author of this book is my father.

My first rotation during internship was hematology-oncology at Brigham and Women's Hospital in Boston. I felt confident enough; after all, I had been studying and preparing for this moment for 4 years. I inherited quite a service, including four women under the age of 40 with advanced non-Hodgkin lymphoma. The outgoing intern smiled with relief as he signed out to me, adding that the sickest of these young women was the favorite patient of the chief of the division. As he left, he simply added, "I wouldn't let her die on your watch if I were you."

Needless to say, this young woman began to deteriorate with worsening respiratory failure my first night on call. I reviewed the differential diagnosis in my head: pneumonia because she was immunosupressed, pneumothorax or hemothorax from the internal jugular line that had been placed for access, transfusion-related acute lung injury from the platelets she had received earlier, congestive heart failure from fluid overload or chemotherapy-induced cardiomyopathy, or even pulmonary embolus given her sedentary status. A brief perusal of my *Washington Manual* bolstered these thoughts, and I ordered a stat chest x-ray.

That is when the panic really began to set in. I would have to interpret and act on that chest x-ray ... was I really prepared for this? I had always been comfortable in the x-ray department, as I had spent significant time in my childhood following my father around while he read films, but I had had little formal training. Radiology wasn't an individual requirement of my medical school curriculum; it was assumed you would be exposed to it during your clinical rotations. I had even taken the elective in radiology, but this actually consisted of simply sitting in an empty reading room reviewing chest films from case studies in the film library, on my own. Yet now I was on the front line caring for a sick woman and would have to implement the appropriate therapy based on my interpretation of the film.

So what were my resources? My resident was tied up with an admission in the emergency room. The radiology resident would give me a quick read when he had time, but he was busy with another procedure. The radiology attending wouldn't over-read the film until the morning. The clinical scenario demanded an immediate decision on therapy, so I would have to try my best to interpret the film.

My experience that night led to the first of many conversations with my father regarding the status of radiology education in our medical training. Given the explosion of diagnostic imaging we use and rely on every day in the care of our patients, change would be imperative. Since that time, great strides have certainly been made. In many medical schools, imaging studies are now fully integrated into many courses such as anatomy; my father pioneered just such an initiative at UConn. Other schools have now added radiology requirements to their core curricula. Nevertheless, we still have a way to go. Standardization of basic curriculum requirements remains lacking. Many medical schools have shifted their training focus to outpatient settings, where direct interaction with diagnostic imaging is less likely—you will certainly review the report but not necessarily the imaging itself. And there is a growing component of care provided by physician extenders—PAs, NPs, and RNs—whose background training in reading even the most basic of radiology imaging is even less rigorous.

Why wasn't there a radiology equivalent to the *Washington Manual* that could help care providers get through a night like the one I had? It made perfect sense, but I could find no resource like this available. I jokingly referred to my idea as "Lines, Tubes, and

Drains: Radiology for Dummies." But once I discussed it with my father, it was no joke: A new project was born. It has grown and evolved over time, but he has worked tirelessly and diligently to bring a radiology reference manual aimed at providers on the front line of care to fruition. As we rely ever increasingly on imaging, I think this resource will prove invaluable to generations to come. I am extremely proud to introduce this new effort of my father, and I hope it fulfills its role for you.

January 21, 2009   Robert Moskowitz, MD

PREFACE

During the past several years, there have been very few publications concerned with the field of ICU radiology. The portable chest x-ray has always been, and still is, one of the most important parts of the work up and treatment of a patient in the ICU. The film provides a reflection of the hemodynamics and an assessment of the etiology of the pathology of each patient. While the rest of radiology has enjoyed incredible change due to technological innovation and improvement, the ICU portable is still performed with equipment that has not changed over the past 30–40 years and is probably the least technologically advanced piece of equipment in the radiologic armamentarium. While the portable film can be augmented by other sophisticated studies, such as CT and MRI, moving the patient to obtain these studies is often extremely difficult and, at times, impossible. In effect, the portable film serves as a screening device as well as a diagnostic tool for the treatment of these very sick patients.

The material in this book stems from my experience as a radiologist at the University of Connecticut Health Center, where I reviewed all of the ICU films each day with the ICU team. At the urging of my students, ICU radiology became a mini-course that I taught during the 4th-year radiology elective.

This book is not intended to be a major reference source but is, in effect, an introduction to the way a student or a resident can approach and read an ICU film. It is a reflection of my own approach and philosophy toward x-ray interpretation of the ICU patient. The method proposed is one I use daily and one that can be used in any ICU setting. An attempt has been made to maintain a straightforward, orderly, and practical format and to emphasize specific points that I have found to be useful and that often can make a difference in a patient's management. The most common problems are covered in detail and most rare ones are dealt with only superficially or not at all.

Interpreting a portable ICU film demands considerable art mixed with a limited amount of science, but understanding the underlying pathology and hemodynamics is extremely important and helpful and provides a sound foundation for the meaningful interpretation of the film. One must also look at many films because experience is a great teacher, and this takes time; thus this book can serve only as a starting point.

Section I of the book is divided into 10 chapters, starting with a short discussion of the physics necessary to obtain a proper film and proceeding to such topics as malalignment of tubes and lines, barotrauma, pneumonia and air-space diseases, congestive failure. Section II of the book consists of additional cases pertaining to each chapter. The cases are also included on the accompanying CD. After reading each chapter, students can test themselves with these cases, and then listen as I discuss the pertinent findings on the film. I hope this will enable readers to obtain considerable experience in recognizing common problems.

I would like to thank the many people who have had a hand in helping me with this book. First and foremost, I would like to acknowledge that the inspiration for this book sprang from my son Rob's experience as a medical student and resident and his recognition of the need for students and residents to have a primer in how to approach the ICU portable in the middle of the night. Then I would like to thank the many 4th-year students and residents who have taken my radiology course and helped me shape and learn how to present this material, so that they could be successful in reading films. I am indebted to my colleagues on the front line, those in the ICU, who taught me and helped find the cases I use both in this textbook and in everyday teaching.

I am indebted to Martha Wilke for helping initiate the laborious typing of this manuscript and Jennifer Clark Evans who has typed, and retyped, the manuscript with grace and dedication. I salute my many friends and family who have lent encouragement and I would like to recognize my wife, Janet, who has diligently edited this book. Finally, I would like to acknowledge my debt to Andrew Warren who has worked tirelessly and long in digitizing the many images that appear within. My grateful appreciation to all.

HAROLD MOSKOWITZ, MD

PRINCIPLES

CHAPTER 1

INTRODUCTION

Patients in the ICU are the most critically ill patients in the hospital. They are usually supported by many different types of mechanical devices and generally have many monitoring lines, tubes, and catheters. Critical management of these patients can change from minute to minute. Physicians depend on the physical examination of their patients, which is often quite difficult, and the portable chest radiograph to help understand the patient's problems. While CT and ultrasound can be of enormous help with these sick patients, the portable chest radiograph is the most helpful and most commonly used x-ray examination. The malposition of lines, tubes, and catheters and cardiopulmonary complications, such as atelectasis, pneumonia, failure, and effusions, are often initially detected on the portable film.

One of the more frightening experiences for a 1st-year resident is to be summoned to the ICU in the middle of the night as the result of a marked deterioration of a patient. A portable chest x-ray is generally obtained, which reveals a plethora of tubes, lines, and

ICU Chest Radiology: Principles and Case Studies, by Harold Moskowitz
Copyright © 2010 John Wiley & Sons, Inc.

mechanical-assist devices as well as a multitude of cardiopulmonary problems manifested in many different guises. Compounding the problem is the fact that a portable film often does not have the technical quality of films obtained in the radiology department, and there is no radiologist available to help the resident make important life-deciding decisions.

Very little attention has been paid to teaching medical students, residents, and ICU nurses how to approach and read an ICU film. The purpose of this book is to address the more common problems a student will encounter. Attention to the issues and clinical problems that are displayed herein should provide the student with the framework for intelligent and, I hope, accurate interpretation of the changes seen on chest film found in these patients. This book should help the student identify and correct any abnormal positions in the various devices inserted into the vascular and respiratory systems and identify abnormalities of the cardiopulmonary system.

The book consists of a series of chapters discussing various issues, including how to obtain a proper film and the more common clinical problems encountered each day in an ICU. The accompanying CD has one to nine cases relating to the topics covered in each chapter. Cases are presented that simulate common problems in the ICU. Each case has a short clinical history followed by a portable radiograph. Each case is the result of a sudden change in a patient's condition, which resulted in an x-ray being obtained. The reader is encouraged to look at the radiograph, identify the various problems, determine the clinical condition that caused the deterioration in the patient, and plan what to do about the problems discussed. I have been teaching this course as part of the 4th-year radiology elective at the University of Connecticut Health Center for 5 years. As I explain the situation to the students, it is 2:00 A.M. and the nurse in the ICU has just awakened you to tell you that one of your patients has crashed. The reader tells the nurse to get a chest radiograph and arrives 5 minutes later in the ICU. What do you see and what are you planning to do about it? That is the name of the game.

After studying at the radiograph, the student should turn to the discussion of the findings, which includes an interpretation of the problems found and an outline of the course of action to be followed. It is hoped that this will help the reader solidify the concepts presented in Section I of the book.

CHAPTER 2

PORTABLE CHEST TECHNIQUE IN THE ICU

The portable chest radiograph is the most common test used at the bedside to evaluate the cardiopulmonary status of patients in the ICU. On the portable film, one can detect the positions of lines, tubes, and monitoring devices as well as evaluate the patient's disease status and response to therapy.[1]

Careful attention should be given to the technique used in obtaining a chest radiograph. The quality of the portable radiography is often highly variable and generally inferior to examinations performed in the main department. Poor technical quality of a portable chest radiograph may result in a delay or the inability to establish a diagnosis. Because of the portable film's necessity and its variable quality, it is important for the reader to understand, and keep in mind, several important differences between routine chest films obtained in the x-ray department and those obtained portably.[2]

A portable chest radiograph is often of inferior quality because of (1) the difficulty controlling scattered radiation, (2) the wide range of densities that need to be demonstrated on a film, and (3) the inability of critically ill patients to cooperate. Furthermore, the

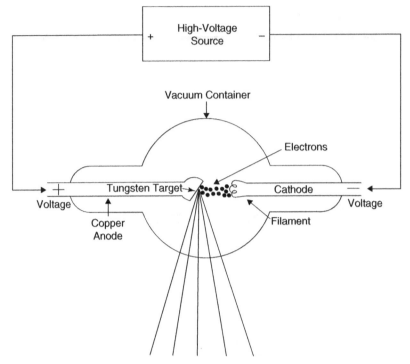

Figure 2.1   An x-ray tube.

portable machine is one of the most inefficient and technically least advanced pieces of imaging equipment in an x-ray department (Fig. 2.1).[3]

A team approach is needed to obtain a portable chest radiograph, and the team should include technologists, radiologists, and ICU personnel. There should be close cooperation between ICU nurses, respiratory therapists, and other ICU personnel in assisting the technologist while positioning an unstable patient. They should help remove unnecessary and unwanted tubes and lines from the patient's chest before taking the film because these can be misinterpreted and thought to be in the heart or lungs. Furthermore, every attempt must be made to obtain the film with the patient upright and at the end of deep inspiration. If the radiograph is obtained in expiration when the patient is supine, the findings can be misleading. Finally, it is imperative that there be rapid communication between the radiologist and the ICU team about the findings seen on a chest radiograph.[4]

Because the quality of the image often determines the diagnostic information that can be obtained from the radiograph, it is necessary to review the factors affecting the film, such as contrast, noise, and spatial resolution.

Contrast represents the variation of film density between one part of the film and another. Ideally one should obtain a film with the highest contrast throughout, and in the chest x-ray this is generally measured from the darkest area (D_{max}), which is the lung, to the lightest, white area (D_{min}), which is bone. Contrast is the result of the differences between tissues as an x-ray photon passes through the object. The important parameters are thickness and density of the material through which the x-ray passes and the amount of absorption of the photon that occurs. In the diagnostic radiology range ($60–150\,KV_p$) the absorption coefficient has a direct relationship to the atomic number of the tissue through which the photon passes. In this range, the absorption coefficient is related to the cube of the atomic number. Objects with a high atomic number have a different contrast resolution than do objects with a lower atomic number. This permits us to differentiate structures because in the chest x-ray the heart has a different density, and a different atomic number, than the surrounding lung. The ribs and bony structures are made up principally of calcium, which has a higher atomic number than the lung and thus absorbs more of the x-ray beam, and are therefore easily visualized.[5]

Noise degrades an image. It is generally seen as grainy mottle pattern on the x-ray. This is due to the statistical difference in the number of x-ray photons striking the film in different areas. In some areas, there are insufficient numbers of photons, so only a part of the film is exposed, producing a mottled appearance.

Spatial resolution is the ability of an x-ray to depict closely spaced objects. High spatial resolution produces sharper edges in an object than does low resolution. Image sharpness refers to how sharp the edge of an object is when seen adjacent to other objects.[6]

The key to optimizing the technical quality of a chest radiograph is to minimize variation in the technical parameters from day to day. One should instruct the technologist to choose the same patient position each day and to keep a written record of the previous successful techniques at each patient's bedside. The first time a film is obtained on an ICU patient, the technologist should show that film to the ICU radiologist, who will determine if the technique is adequate. If so, this technique should subsequently be used on all follow-up films so that the exposure is similar and changes in the most recent x-ray are due to changes in the patient's condition, rather than changes induced by differences in radiologic technique.[7]

It is necessary to keep in mind that portable chest films are performed in the anterior posterior (AP) position, resulting in a 15–20% magnification factor to the cardiac shadow. One should be cautious when making the diagnosis of cardiomegaly on an AP film. Remember that one needs an adequate inspiration (9–10 ribs) to establish that diagnosis.[8]

Exposure variations constitute one of the main difficulties in portable radiography. Photo-timing devices, used in the main department, are generally not used for bedside films.[9] Generally, the exposure must be estimated by the technologist. The principal variables that affect quality film include the kilovolt potential (KV_p) and milliampere second (mAs) used, the patient's size, the use of a grid, the film system speed, and the distance between the x-ray tube and the image receptor.

While it is possible to vary the kVp setting, this is normally not done because altering the kVp even minimally will produce large changes in exposure. On a portable chest film, a 20% change in kVp will be the equivalent of doubling the mAs.

The mAs is the product of tube current in milliamperes (mA) and exposure time in seconds (s). Normally the mA is fixed, and change occurs due to variations made in the time of exposure. Generally, the technologist adjusts the mAs to achieve correct film exposure.

Thus normally the kVp is kept constant and the mAs is varied. If the distance between tube and film is increased, the mAs needs to be increased. Increasing the mAs poses a problem especially in large patients or those who are unable to hold their breath because lack of sharpness occurs on exposure times greater than 10 ms.

Patient size is another variable, but an experienced technologist can quickly estimate the need for increased exposure when needed. The degree of pathology in the lung also contributes to the necessity for increasing exposure because abnormalities that increase density in the lung cause more of the x-ray beam to be absorbed.

In portable radiography, the distance between the x-ray tube and the film is not fixed. It is extremely important to keep tube–film distance unchanged from day to day. Exposure is inversely related to distance, so small variations in distance can account for large changes in exposure. A change of 6 in. from one day to the next can result in a 50% variance in film exposure; 50 in. is the optimal distance from tube to film.

Portable radiographs are of inferior quality mainly because of the amount of scattered radiation that occurs during a routine portable chest film.[10] When an x-ray beam passes through a patient, the resulting exit beam contains both primary and scattered radiation. The primary radiation consists of photons of energy that proceed directly through a patient to strike the film and produce an image. Scatter refers to photons that have changed direction and then strike the film, producing an image. There is, however, no diagnostic information obtained because the direction of these photons is totally random and cannot be interpreted. Scatter results in loss of contrast as well as loss of resolution resulting in a degradation of quality.[11] This can lead to films in which important information, such as the location of catheters and mediastinal abnormalities, are difficult to evaluate. Scatter can be reduced by the use of a grid. Grids are made of thin, flat strips of lead running parallel to each other with plastic inlays between them. This grid is placed between the patient and the film. The lead strips absorb all but the directly parallel photons and thus all scatter is absorbed, improving the quality of the film (Fig. 2.2).

Using a grid results in remarkable cleanup of the scatter on a film, and it is surprising that many hospitals fail to routinely use a grid for their portable ICU films. There are two principle objections to the use of grids. One is the physical burden; the grid is heavy and technologists must carry this as well as the cassette. The second objection is that in order to obtain a proper film, the grid must be properly aligned with the x-ray beam, which may be a difficult task. Improper alignment can result in a poor film due to grid cutoff. Grid cutoff occurs when the grid is not centered and is improperly placed with respect to the x-ray beam. This results in the lead lines of the grid absorbing most, or a significant portion, of the beam, producing a light film.[12] A 6:1 or 8:1 grid will improve film quality significantly and should be routinely used. A linear 6:1 grid combined with a

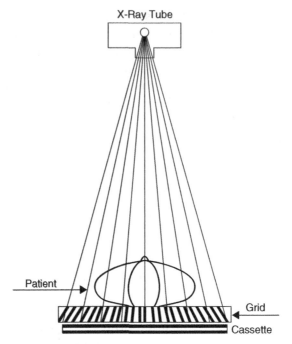

Figure 2.2   A 5:1 grid.

wide-latitude film screen should produce a film of excellent quality, with good contrast between the lung and the mediastinal areas.

Failure to use a grid permits large amounts of scatter to strike the film, resulting in loss of contrast and inability to produce a film of diagnostic quality. Scatter is most pronounced in the denser areas of the chest, such as the mediastinum. Some people express the amount of scatter radiation as the *scatter fraction*, which is defined as the ratio of scattered radiation to total radiation. In portable ICU radiography, the scatter fraction varies but may be as high as 95%, indicating that scatter constitutes 95% of the radiation recorded by the film, thus severely degrading the image and delivering a considerable amount of unnecessary radiation to the patient.

The conventional grid consists of a series of closely placed strips of lead. Often it is referred to as a *Bucky*, after the work of Gustav Bucky, who published his work in 1939. His design is still the basic configuration used today. The ratio between the height of the strips and the spaces between them is referred to as the grid ratio

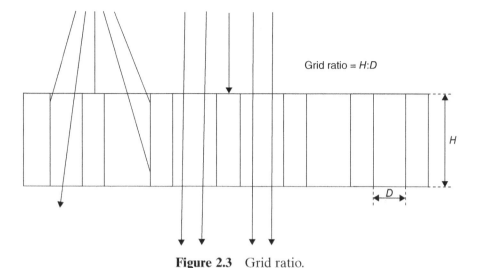

Figure 2.3   Grid ratio.

(Fig. 2.3), which is the most important consideration for grid perfor-
mance. There are several common variations of grids: focused versus
parallel grid strips, and linear versus cross-hatched grids. In a focused
grid, the strips converge slightly toward the center, so the transmis-
sion of the primary x-ray beam can be equal across the entire width
of the grid. This feature is very important when imaging large areas
such as the chest, especially at the short distance used in portable
radiography. A linear strip grid has the unique advantage of being
sensitive to alignment in only one plane. Angulation across the direction of the grid causes grid cutoff, but angulation along the direction
of the gridline produces no loss of image quality. The grids generally
used in portable chest radiography are of the linear strip type, and
the technologist need be concerned only with alignment in a single
plane.

The *angle of acceptance* is the angle whereby noticeable cutoff will
occur when one angles the tube across the linear relationship of the
lead grid lines. The ideal grid should provide excellent scatter control
and have a wide angle of acceptance. Unfortunately, these qualities
are fundamentally incompatible. The higher the grid ratio, the more
complete the scatter rejection; however, the angle of acceptance is
very small. For most work in the ICU using 80–90 kVp, an 8:1 grid
is an effective compromise. Higher grid ratios, such as 12:1, may

provide better scatter cleanup but have significant inherent difficulties in their use.

Various types of specialized grids were developed approximately 10 years ago for use in ICU radiology, but they have largely been supplanted by the use of digital radiography in which only an external grid can be used.

In previous decades, chemical processing had to be discussed at great length, but with today's digital and computer radiography techniques, this issue is no longer significant in most radiology departments. Improper processing was a major cause of inferior image quality. However, the issues of automatic processing, temperature control, sensitometric film strips, and developer solutions as well as the fogging of film are no longer of major concern.

The clinician must always remember that portable chest x-rays subject the patient to a radiation dose 2–4 times that of a radiograph made on standard equipment in an x-ray department. Most ICUs are concerned that scattered radiation may constitute a health hazard to nurses and other ancillary personnel.

In two new separate studies, however, there was no significant radiation exposure to ICU personnel from portable chest radiographs.[13]

Digital radiography has rapidly gained acceptance for ICU portable chest x-rays. Storage phosphor-computed radiography is the method used in almost all hospitals ICUs.[14] A plate coated with photostimulable phosphor material is used instead of film to record the image. The plate is contained in a rigid cassette similar to those used in conventional film systems. Interaction of an x-ray photon with the phosphor produces a latent image of trapped electrons in the phosphor material. The quantity of trapped electrons is proportional to the incident x-ray intensity. After it has been exposed, the cassette is placed in the processor, which unloads the exposed plate and replaces it with an erased one. A finely focused laser beam scans the plate, causing the trapped energy to be released as light, which is recorded and converted to a digital signal.[15] This digital signal can be recorded on a film or can be entered into a picture-archiving computerized system (PACS).[16] An advantage to digital radiography is the wide latitude of the recording system, which allows an excellent image over a wide range of exposure. This technique is thus more forgiving than conventional radiography, an advantage that is most apparent when one has to x-ray ICU patients because over-exposure or underexposure, which is frequent with routine films, can be all but eliminated. The wide dynamic range, as well as the ability to postprocess the image, helps improve visualization of the lungs, tubes, and mediastinal structures. There are also new types of algorithms that decrease the effect of scatter. Disadvantages of this technique are higher image noise and lower spatial resolution and some increased dose. This technique was first developed by Fuji Corporation and marketed by Philips. True digital imaging is hard to use in the ICU because its receptor cannot be moved from patient to patient.

The major reason storage phosphor imaging was applied to portables was to achieve consistent reproduction of an image. Contrast is increased, and there is often improved image quality through the thicker parts of the chest due to image processing. An important consideration when using computerized radiography is that computerized radiography plates are more susceptible to degradation by scatter than are conventional systems, due to their relatively higher sensitivity to low-energy radiation. It is important then, to note that the use of a grid will have a greater impact on a computer radiography system for portable chest radiographs than on conventional systems. Also remember that the use of a grid requires increased exposure for the patients.

A digital radiograph is one in which the image has been divided into a matrix of discrete picture elements (pixels), each of which is assigned a specific value. Once digitized, the image can be stored, transmitted, reproduced, or manipulated to enhance diagnostic details. The pixel size is determined by the size of the area imaged and the digital matrix used. Up to a point, the smaller the pixel size, the better the image quality. Most radiologists suggest that a pixel size of 0.2 mm or smaller is necessary to achieve a level of diagnostic accuracy comparable to that of conventional radiography.

The advantages of combining a digital system with PACS include (1) more consistent acquisition of diagnostic radiographs; (2) the ability to manipulate images by adjusting window levels and settings; (3) the ability to rapidly transmit images over computer networks so they may be viewed simultaneously by the radiologist and the consulting physician; (4) the ability of the radiologist to use tools such as scrolling, image navigation, and window and level measurements;

and (5) the ability to find the location of tubes and catheters and facilitate measuring areas of tissue density in the patient. PACS also allows for instant reconstruction of several planes of the image.[17]

The integration of a hospital information system (HIS) with a PACS and a voice-recognition reporting system, has streamlined the flow of information between ICU physicians and radiologists. Physician order entry also helps by giving the referring physician an opportunity to provide essential clinical information to aid selection of appropriate studies. It also provides the radiologist with instant clinical data to aid in protocolling studies and help in interpretation.

Many years ago, most radiology departments struggled to offer prompt, reliable access to the portable chest x-rays obtained in the ICU. Films would be lost or misplaced, and occasionally this delay would result in missing important findings. Digital imaging and the use of a PACS system have eliminated this problem completely.

The introduction and use of computerized radiography and PACS have transformed the interaction between radiology and the ICU.[18] PACS are composed of image-acquisition systems and network display devices as well as storage devices. Images used for interpretation by radiologists are viewed on high-resolution monitors, and one can simultaneously review or send images among several remote sites. One may look at and transmit images not only of the chest but of any part of the body via this system. Images should be reviewed on high-resolution monitors because finding abnormalities, such as a small pneumothorax, can be difficult on low-quality monitors.

Although this instant access to the radiology image is helpful to the ICU physician, it is important that there still be daily direct communication between the radiologist and the ICU clinician. PACS has decreased the direct communication between radiologists and the clinician. With the ability to view x-rays directly in the ICU, clinicians often do not consult with the radiologist after reviewing the images themselves. This declining communication between the clinician and the radiologist may have a negative impact on patient care. It is important for the clinician to review a film with the radiologist before going ahead with a significant clinical action.

Team conferences and rounds with the radiologist can facilitate communication and provide an explanation for any findings on the portable chest x-ray.

CHAPTER 3

APPROACH TO READING A PORTABLE CHEST RADIOGRAPH

It is important to remember when reading a chest film that you are responsible for *all* findings on the x-ray, not simply those associated with the heart and lungs. For this reason, a systematic approach should be developed and used each and every time a film is reviewed. In this way important and even unrelated findings will not go unrecognized.

Obviously, the first thing to do is to determine that the film you are reviewing is of the correct patient and was done at the particular time and date for which you are interested. This is important because critically ill patients in the ICU may have had several films taken in a 24-hour time span.

The first evaluation one must make is to determine the technical quality of the film. The reader must ask and answer this important question: Is the technique adequate so that the film can be read? The three most important parameters that must be reviewed are

1. Is there rotation of the patient?
2. Is the exposure of the film adequate?
3. Is the inspiratory effort of the patient adequate?

ICU Chest Radiology: Principles and Case Studies, by Harold Moskowitz
Copyright © 2010 John Wiley & Sons, Inc.

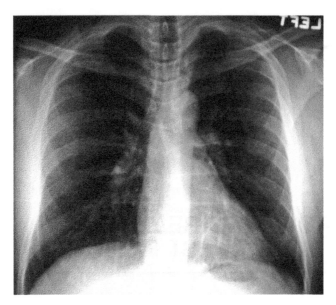

Figure 3.1   A normal portable x-ray without rotation, adequately exposed, and in deep inspiration.

Rotation can simulate abnormalities in the cardiac contour or in the mediastinal shadow, which can lead to erroneous diagnoses (Fig. 3.1). To determine whether a film is centered, check the position of the medial ends of the clavicles in relation to the spinous process of the spine. If the clavicles are not equidistant from the spinous process, the patient is rotated. If the left clavicle is closer to the spinous process, then the patient is rotated into the left anterior oblique position. If the right clavicle is closer to the spinous process, then the patient is in the right anterior oblique position. One can also determine the degree of rotation by measuring on each side, from the edge of the thoracic spine to the edge the rib cage on that side, and comparing it to the other side. If they measure the same, there is no significant rotation.

Next, the reader must determine whether the film is adequately exposed. Underpenetration can increase or even create the appearance of alveolar densities, and overpenetration can burn through similar alveolar densities so that they are not appreciated. One can judge the degree of penetration by evaluating how well the thoracic vertebrae are seen through the heart shadow. In a properly exposed

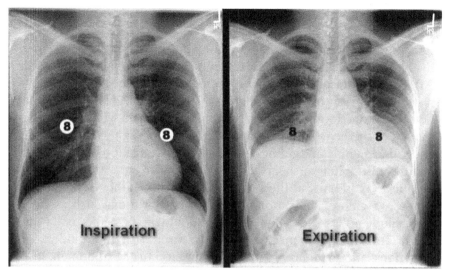

Figure 3.2   These films reveal the significant changes in heart size and pulmonary volume that occur during inspiration and expiration.

film, one should just be able to make out the thoracic vertebrae and also be able to look through the cardiac shadow to see structures in the left lower lobe of the lung, especially the lower lobe vasculature.

The third evaluation a reader must make is to determine whether the film has been taken in adequate inspiration (Fig. 3.2). Expiratory films can often mislead the reader into thinking there are densities and infiltrates in the lower lobes. An expiratory film may also mislead the reader into misinterpreting the size of the cardiac shadow. If the patient has taken an adequate inspiration, the right hemidiaphragm should be at approximately the 9th or 10th rib when counting the posterior ribs. Sometimes it is difficult to count the upper ribs on the right. Start by finding the anterior portion of the 1st and then the 2nd rib (the anterior ribs can almost always be seen). Trace the 2nd rib back and find the 2nd rib posteriorly. Count down. When the right hemidiaphragm is at the 11th or 12th rib, the patient probably has chronic obstructive pulmonary disease (COPD).

Remember, if the film is not technically adequate the reader should request that the technologist return and get an adequate film. This will permit an accurate interpretation, and you will not be misled by poor technique.

SYSTEMATIC REVIEW

Each individual must develop a routine that is carefully and repetitively followed each time one reviews a portable chest radiograph. After the technical aspects have been evaluated one should begin a systematic review of everything that is on the film. My recommendation is that one look at the heart and lungs last. You will never forget to look at the heart and lungs on a chest radiograph, while you may miss other significant findings if you get involved in looking at abnormalities of the lung or heart.

Thus look initially at the soft tissues; starting in the neck, look for masses, vascular calcification, and other calcifications such as calcified lymph nodes. Next, look at the shoulders, past the axilla and down into the abdomen. In the axilla, search for lymph nodes, calcifications, and evidence of previous surgery. In the abdomen, look for free air, intestinal obstruction, and calcifications. Note the presence of grafts, renal or gallstones, and abnormal soft tissue masses.

One should then proceed to look at the bony structures. Look first at the neck and the cervical vertebral column. Then carefully evaluate both clavicles, both scapula, and the shoulders. Each rib should be looked at individually. It is important to go from posterior to anterior, visualizing each portion of the rib: the cortex, the medulla, its junction with the costal cartilage and the vertebral column. The thoracic vertebrae and para-vertebral soft tissues should be evaluated. Look at the vertebral bodies' spinous processes, transverse processes, lamina, pedicles, and articulating vertebral facets. Also, carefully evaluate both diaphragms and the costophrenic sulcus to resolve the question of fluid before turning attention to the lung fields.

It is recommended that viewing and comparing the lung fields be done in thirds: upper, middle, and lower lung fields. Each hilum should be individually evaluated; consider the size of each hilum and the pulmonary arteries. Are the pulmonary veins and bronchi normal? Is there any evidence of pulmonary hypertension or adenopathy? The costophrenic sulci should be evaluated to determine if there is fluid or whether the angle is blunted. Is there any loss of volume? Check for a shift of mediastinum or of the fissures. Are there any abnormal densities, fibrosis, or air bronchograms?

Attention should then turn to the cardiac border. Evaluate cardiac size and potential chamber enlargement. Remember too, that this is a portable film, generally performed at 50 in. It is usually thought that the heart is enlarged when it measures more than 50% of the transverse width of the chest. This is somewhat misleading on portable films since there is a 15–20% magnification factor. Still, overall, one can usually use 50% as a fairly accurate determination of cardiac enlargement. One can measure the width of the heart and compare it to thoracic width to see if it approximates 50%, or one can use a technique that I have found useful. In a properly exposed film in adequate inspiration and without rotation, pick up the portion of the cardiac shadow from the edge of the right vertebral border to the heart border. Visualize in your mind's eye taking it to the left heart border. If it touches the rib cage the heart is enlarged. The right atrium, ascending aorta, vascular pedicle, arch of the aorta, pulmonary artery, left atrial appendage, and left ventricular borders should all be evaluated. Are there any calcifications in the aorta, cardiac valve area, or coronary arteries? Do you see signs of ventricular aneurysms?

Also, carefully review the current film and compare it to the previous one, if available. Changes in a patient's condition occur rapidly, and one must always determine if there has been worsening or improvement of a patient's condition in order to change or persist in current therapy.

Only with this systematic approach to the evaluation of a chest radiograph will you recognize all the abnormalities you are responsible for finding on your patient's film.

CHAPTER 4

TUBES, LINES AND CATHETERS

The ICU patient is unique in that he or she is in critical or unstable condition and requires a great deal of medical care. Most of these patients have either undergone major surgery (e.g., cardiac surgery), had serious trauma, have overwhelming infection, or have failure of one or more organ systems.

Because of their serious condition, most patients in the ICU are monitored by many different types of tubes, lines, and catheters. Malposition of these devices can be life threatening. A portable chest radiograph is almost always obtained following placement or manipulation of any of these devices to evaluate its position (Fig. 4.1). It is very important to be able to identify not only the type of device in place but also its correct position, as malposition will often complicate and potentially lead to the deterioration of the patient's condition.[19]

ENDOTRACHEAL TUBE

Many patients are treated for respiratory failure and thus a patent airway and adequate oxygenation are critical components of their

ICU Chest Radiology: Principles and Case Studies, by Harold Moskowitz
Copyright © 2010 John Wiley & Sons, Inc.

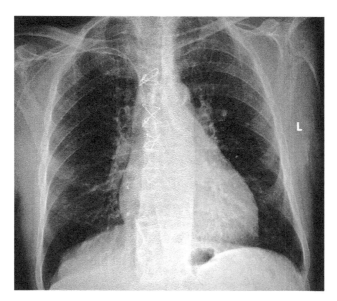

Figure 4.1   A normal postoperative film of a patient with mild to moderate cardiomegaly.

care. There are many problems that lead to endotracheal intubation. Among these are failure of the patient to have adequate gas exchange, the possibility of airway obstruction, and an attempt to provide airway protection. Any one of these conditions will lead to the placement of an endotracheal tube (ETT). A positive-pressure mechanical ventilator is most often attached to the endotracheal tube. Chest x-rays are indicated after intubation to ensure the proper position of the tube and to check for possible complications (Fig. 4.2). An ETT can be placed by an oral or a nasal route, but the most important consideration is to check the position of the tip of the tube in relation to the carina.[20]

In patients with respiratory failure, a positive-pressure mechanical ventilator is generally used, and this requires placement of an ETT. A portable chest x-ray is obtained to determine whether the endotracheal tube is in proper position (Fig. 4.3). The ideal position for the tube is in the mid-trachea, approximately 4 cm above the carina.[20,21]

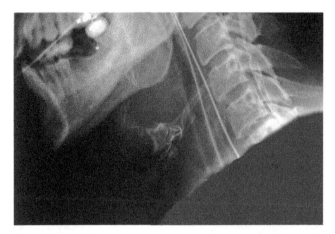

Figure 4.2 A lateral film of the neck reveals the normal position of a nasaogastric tube posterior to the endotracheal tube.

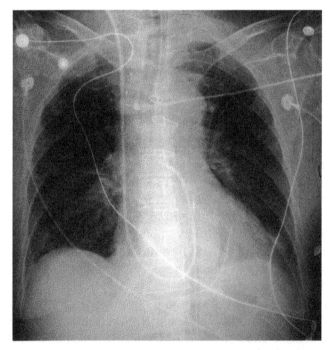

Figure 4.3 A portable x-ray reveals good position of the ETT approximately 4cm above carina. Note the intra-aorta balloon pump in mid-dorsal aorta.

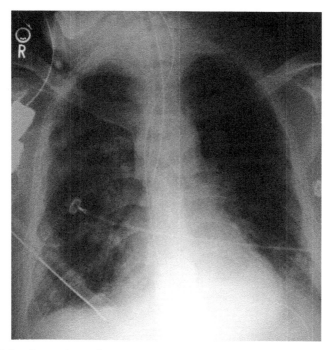

Figure 4.4 An endotracheal tube in the right main stem bronchus caused by the patient flexing his head, which moves the tube downward.

This distance from the carina has been shown to be optimal because it allows a safe margin if the head is maximally flexed, which could drive the ET tube downward, or if the patient extends his head, elevating the tube. Proper placement of the tube will prevent it from either riding too high or slipping down, generally into the right main stem bronchus, resulting in inadequate ventilation of the left lung (Fig. 4.4).[22]

The carina is identified by tracing the left main stem bronchus back to its junction with the right main stem bronchus.

When the carina can not be visualized on the radiograph, one can estimate its position by identifying the T4–T5 interspace, which generally indicates the location of the carina. Improper placement, if undetected, can cause hyperinflation and possibly pneumothorax of the intubated side. If an endotracheal tube is not advanced far enough, inadvertent extubation can occur or the tube could

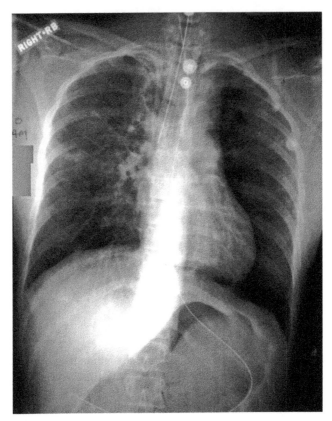

Figure 4.5   The cuff on the endotracheal tube is overinflated, which may cause ischemia of the tracheal mucosa.

ride up high enough to put the vocal cords at risk.[23] One can visualize the endotracheal tube by visualizing the thin radio opaque line along its length.

The cuff of the endotracheal tube should be inflated sufficiently to occlude the airway but should never exceed the width of the trachea. If one visualizes a bulge in the tracheal wall, this indicates overinflation of the balloon, which can result in damage to the tracheal mucosa, with secondary complications such as ulceration and stricture (Fig. 4.5).[24]

One must be alert to the possible malposition of the endotracheal tube into the pharynx, resulting in aspiration and vocal cord damage.

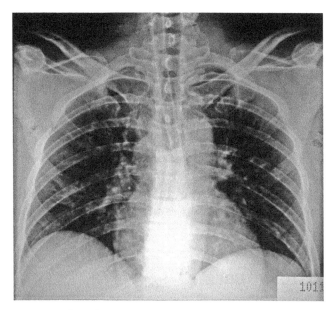

Figure 4.6 Note that the endotracheal tube is not within lumen of the trachea but rather in the esophagus.

Esophogeal intubation, another complication, can be recognized by the overdistention of the balloon, lateral displacement of the tube relative to the trachea, and overdistention of the stomach (Fig. 4.6).[25]

A very uncommon complication of intubation is tracheal rupture. This probably is related to the use of a stylet; often, the rush of performing the procedure in an emergency results in rapidly apparent subcutaneous emphysema and occasionally pneumothorax.[26]

There has been controversy over whether postintubation and daily films to check the position of the endotracheal tube are necessary. Many studies have revealed that significant malposition of the endotracheal tube is identified approximately 30% of the time. Based on current available data, a postintubation chest x-ray is indicated for nearly all patients undergoing translaryngeal intubation.[27]

The long-term complications of a patient who is intubated include a high risk of sinusitis, atelectasis, and various types of infections. Intubated patients are also at risk for significant barotrauma. Even aspiration pneumonia can occur in intubated patients because secretions and gastric aspirate can accumulate above the cuff of the endo-tracheal tube and make their way into the lower respiratory tract when the cuff is periodically deflated.

It is extremely important for one to be vigilant about the extent and progression of variations in lung volumes and infiltrates when one interprets a chest x-ray on a patient who is on a ventilator. Improvement or deterioration may be more apparent than real. Apparent improvement in pulmonary infiltrates and a decrease in the size of the vascular pedical and of the heart are seen with increasing pressures and increasing tidal volumes delivered by the respirator. An apparent worsening of any infiltrate and mediastinal widening may be related to a decrease in respiratory support and may also be seen after extubation.[28]

TRACHEOSTOMY TUBES

When long-term intubation is required, an ETT will eventually be replaced by a tracheostomy tube. This has several advantages over the ETT tube. First, changes in the position of the head will not affect the tip of the tube. The proper position of the tracheostomy tube is one half to one third the distance between the tracheal stoma and the carina, and its width should be approximately two thirds of the tracheal width. The tracheostomy tube should be within the center of the trachea without either of its edges rubbing against the side walls of the trachea. Malposition may lead to abrasion and secondary erosion of the trachea, resulting in either stricture or possible perforation of the trachea. If a cuff is used, it should hug, but not overdistend, the wall of the trachea.[29]

After performing a tracheostomy, a chest x-ray should be obtained. At that time, one should search for a pneumomediastinum or a pneumothorax. Occasionally, a lateral view is helpful in determining the correct position of the tracheostomy tube.

CENTRAL VENOUS CATHETERS

Central venous catheters are often used in ICU patients to administer medication or intravenous fluids. They are also used to obtain blood for analysis or to measure central venous pressure. Catheters are inserted either in the upper extremity veins (picc lines) proximally, in the subclavian vein, or in the internal jugular vein. The femoral vein is not often used. Triple lumen catheters are used for short-term renal dialysis, and ports are placed in the chest wall of patients requiring repeated doses of chemotherapy or other forms of pharmacotherapy. The superficial and deep veins of the upper arm end up forming the axillary vein, which at the outer border of the 1st rib continues as the subclavian vein. The internal jugular vein joins the subclavian vein to form the brachiocephalic vein.

The left brachiocephalic vein begins behind the sternal end of the left clavicle and runs anterior to the left subclavian and common carotid arteries. It runs retrosternally arches posteriorly and crosses the midline to join the right braciocephalic vein and form the superior vena cava.

Central venous catheters are most often thin, moderately radio-opaque tubes extending centrally from the peripheral sites mentioned. Knowledge of normal venous thoracic anatomy is useful in determining proper catheter placement.

A central venous catheter ideally should be within the superior vena cava, proximal to the right atrium and beyond the most proximal venous valves (Fig. 4.7). These valves are found approximately 1 in. from the end of subclavian and internal jugular veins before they join to form the brachiocephalic vein. Placement of the catheter tip beyond the venous valves is important for an accurate central venous determination. The large caliper of the superior vena cava allows for greater dilution of the many hypertonic or potentially caustic substances administered through the catheter. The ideal position is just above the right atrium and not in the proximal third of the superior vena cava. Central venous catheters located within the proximal third of the superior vena cava are 16 times more likely to thrombus than those in the distal third of the superior vena cava.

The position of the catheter is critical; those that are placed too far distally can enter the right atrium, potentially producing ventricular arrhythmias or even cardiac perforation.[30] Another potential complication that can occur, especially when using the subclavian approach, is a pneumothorax.[31] A chest x-ray should be obtained immediately after placing a central venous line via this route. There

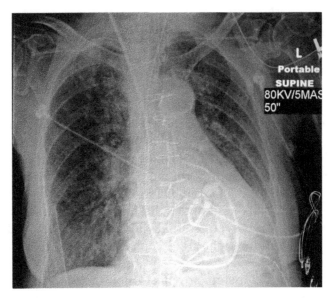

Figure 4.7 The central line is in a good position in the superior vena cava just above the right atrium.

is debate in the literature about whether routine chest radiographs after insertion of central venous catheters are necessary in all patients. Many studies question the value of a chest x-ray's utility because, in competent hands, the number of complications is quite low. Other studies have shown that as many as one third of central venous catheters are not in the correct position on the initial radiograph.

Misplacement of central venous catheters can often be detected on the chest radiograph.[32] On the AP routine chest portable x-ray, subclavian venous catheters should always be behind or inferior to the clavicle. If a radiograph shows a catheter cephalad to the clavicle, one should consider the possibly of intra-arterial or extra-vascular placement.[33] The radiograph should also be assessed for signs of pneumothorax or mediastinal widening, suggesting possible hematoma.[34] Intracardiac placement of a central venous catheter is more common from the right-sided approach than the left sided. Complications include arrhythmias, endothelial damage, and risk of perforation and pericardial tamponade.[35] Occasionally, there may be a peculiar catheter location when the catheter is placed from the

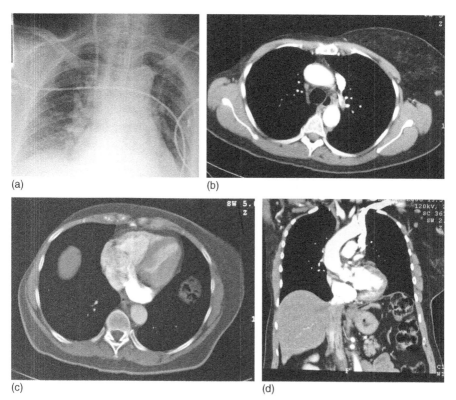

(a)   (b)

(c)   (d)

Figure 4.8   Position of the central line. **A,** The position of the left subclavian line is unusual. **B,** The axial CT reveals contrast in the persistent left superior vena cava. **C,** The axial CT reveals the entrance of the persistent left superior vena cava into the right atrium. **D,** The corporal CT reveals the entire course of the persistent left superior vena cava.

left side. This may be due to the fact that the catheter is in an anomalous vein, occurring in 0.5% of patients. The catheter location can be within a persistent left-sided superior vena cava (Fig. 4.8).[36]

When a catheter is located in the left superior vena cava it mimics an intra-arterial location on the AP radiograph. Occasionally, a catheter can end up in smaller venous side branches, such as the azygos vein.

Infection is a potential complication, especially if the catheter has been in place for longer than 7–10 days. Infection can occur at the

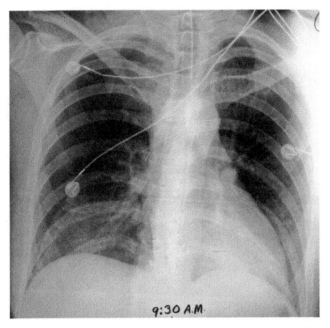

Figure 4.9 A large pneumothrax can be seen on the right, but there is persistent aeration of the right lower lobe.

entry site, and occasionally, mediastinitis and septic emboli can result.[37]

Various studies have shown a 5–7% incidence of pneumothorax after a central line is placed (Fig. 4.9). Always remember that if one is searching for a pneumothorax, an expiratory film should be obtained.[38]

THORACOTOMY TUBES (CHEST TUBES)

Chest tubes are frequently used to evacuate either fluid or air from the pleural space. They consist of a clear plastic tube with side holes and a radio-opaque stripe; a short interruption in this stripe marks the proximal drainage hole. Correct placement of a chest tube depends on whether one wants to evacuate pleural fluid or an empyema or treat a pneumothorax (Fig. 4.10). For a pneumothorax, the tube should be positioned near the lung apex (Fig. 4.11).[39]

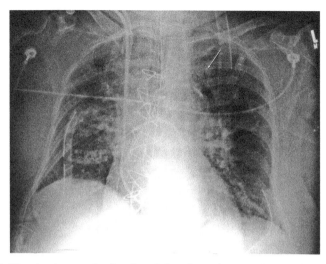

Figure 4.10 A chest tube in the right pleural space. Note the density at the arrow, which was unsuspected bronchogenic carcinoma.

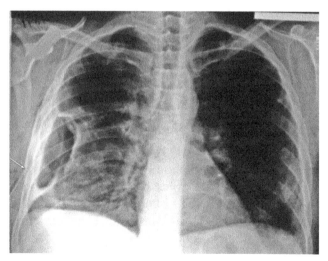

Figure 4.11 The chest tube, identified by the arrow, is seen in the chest wall with associated subcutaneous air. There is a loculated pneumothrax.

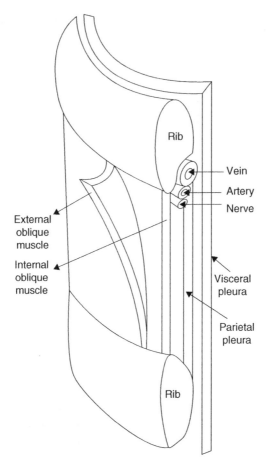

Figure 4.12   The neurovascular bundle at the undersurface of the rib.

To evacuate pleural fluid it should be positioned posteriorly and inferiorly. The proximal side hole should always be medial to the ribs. A film should routinely be obtained after placement of a chest tube. Malfunction of these tubes can result from kinking or debris or from being placed outside the pleura.

One potential complication that can occur at the time of insertion of a chest tube is bleeding due to laceration of an intercostal artery or vein. This injury can be avoided by placing the tube superior to a rib, in order to avoid the neurovascular bundle located at the inferior aspect of the rib (Fig. 4.12).

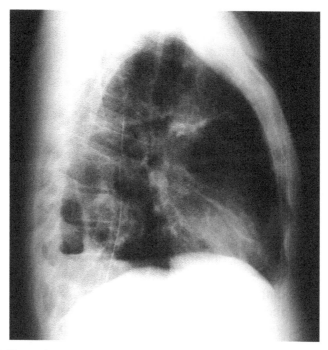

Figure 4.13   A lateral view obtained to reveal the posterior position of the loculated hydropneumothorax.

Malfunction of a tube within a few hours of placement must alert the clinician to the possible misplacement of the tube, perhaps into a fissure.[40]

Placement of a chest tube within a fissure is common and may cause poor function by obstructing drainage. When the chest tube is in the major fissure, the abnormal position may not be appreciated on a frontal radiograph. Think of obtaining a lateral film and one will readily appreciate the tube extending in an oblique orientation along the course of the major fissure (Fig. 4.13). Chest tubes can be advanced too far into the mediastinum or may penetrate into the substance of the lung.[41] Parenchyml placement of the chest tube can lead to intrapulmonary hematomas. Very occasionally, such entities as bronchopulmonary fistula have been reported. These are seen in patients with pleural adhesions or decreased lung compliance.

While a lateral film is often helpful if additional information is needed, a chest CT can be very helpful. Other complications are also easily diagnosed by a chest CT, and it is very helpful for directing the drainage of loculated collections, such as empyema.[42]

NASOGASTRIC TUBES

Nasogastric tubes (NGs), or feeding tubes, are commonly used for suctioning the stomach, feeding the patient, and administering various medications. After placement of an NG tube, a radiograph is important because abnormal position can have serious consequences.[43] Initially, an NG tube should on the left near midline, extending toward the diaphragm.

Once in the stomach, optimal placement depends on whether one is using the tube for feeding or for providing suction in a distended abdomen. Feeding tubes should be placed at least in the gastric antrum or in the duodenum. Distal placement of a feeding tube decreases the possibility of gastroesophageal reflux.

Most nasogastric tubes have multiple side holes extending approximately 10 cm from the distal tip. Therefore, at least 10 cm of tubing should be visualized in the stomach distal to the esophageal gastric junction. If side holes are above the esophageal gastric junction, the possibility of aspiration of gastric contents of tube feedings is significant.

Abnormal positions of a nasogastric tube include the tube being within the tracheobronchial tree or coiled within the pharynx (Fig. 4.14).

These positions also predispose the patient to aspiration. In a large series of cases, 5% of nasogastric tube insertions were in incorrect positions.

Tracheobrochial placement of nasogastric and feeding tubes can cause significant pulmonary complications, including pneumothorax, hydropneumothorax, and extensive aspiration pneumonia. Remember, even in a patient with an endotracheal tube, tracheobronchial placement of a nasogastric tube can occasionally occur.[44] Once in the tracheobronchial system, the tube can actually perforate the lung; we have seen several Dobhoff tubes pierce the lung and end up in the pleural space (Fig. 4.15).[45]

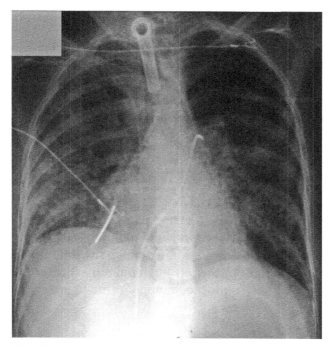

Figure 4.14 Although the patient had a tracheostomy, a Dobhoff tube is seen descending into the right mainstem bronchus and then into the right lower lobe.

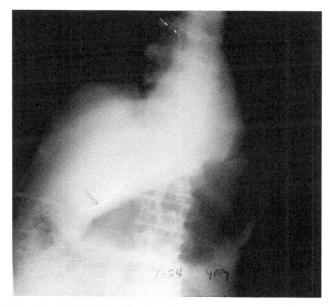

Figure 4.15 The Dobhoff tube has descended into the right lower lung bronchus, perforating the lung and ending up in the posterior pleura space.

Esophageal perforation is a rare but serious complication. The extra esophageal location of an NG tube can be difficult to appreciate on a frontal view and other views, including CT and/or gastrograffin swallow, but may be necessary to establish the diagnosis. X-ray findings include pneumomediastinum, mediastinal widening, and pleural effusion.

SWAN-GANZ CATHETERS

Swan-Ganz catheters (pulmonary artery catheters) are used to measure pulmonary artery pressure, pulmonary capillary wedge pressure, and cardiac output. The catheter tip should normally be within either the right or the left main pulmonary artery (Fig. 4.16). The catheter is inserted most commonly through either the internal

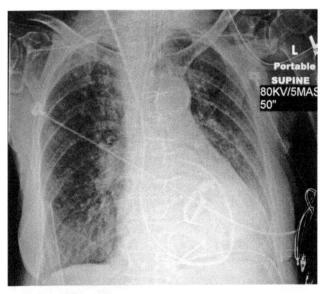

Figure 4.16 A Swan-Ganz catheter is placed from the internal jugular vein, into the right pulmonary artery. The ideal position for this catheter is 3–4 cm distal to the pulmonic valve. Note the prosthetic mitral valve. The endotracheal tube is in good position, as is the nasogastric tube. A chest tube and mediastinal tube are also in good position.

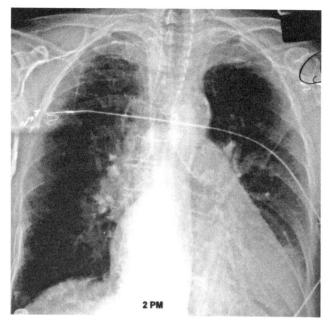

2 PM

Figure 4.17   A portable film taken at 2:00 P.M. reveals normal lung fields with rather large, prominent pulmonary arteries.

jugular or the subclavian route and must not be placed distally into smaller pulmonary vessels (Fig. 4.17).

With inflation of the balloon, the catheter "floats" distally into smaller pulmonary arteries, where a wedge measurement can be obtained. When inflated, the balloon can be seen as 1-cm radiolucency at the tip. When measuring pulmonary wedge pressures, inflate the balloon for only a short period to prevent the possibility of developing pulmonary infarctions. One should never see an inflated balloon on a routine chest radiograph (Fig. 4.18). Thrombus around the catheter can occasionally occur if a catheter is left in place for a prolonged period of time, resulting in possible pulmonary infarcts (Fig. 4.19).[46]

If the catheter tip is placed in the right ventricle or pulmonary outflow tract, arrhythmias or endothelial damage can occur. Another possibility is perforation of the atrium. Arrhythmias and knotting of the catheter are infrequently encountered in clinical practice. A feared complication of the Swan-Ganz catheter is rupture of a small

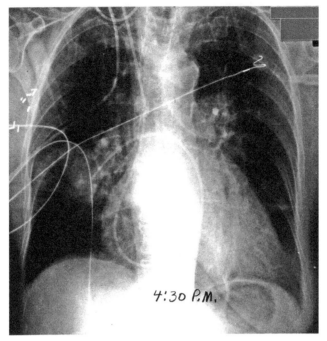

Figure 4.18   A Swan-Ganz catheter was placed distally into the right lung at 4:30 P.M. Note that the balloon is expanded, with a density surrounding the balloon secondary to an area of infarction or hemorrhage.

pulmonary artery, secondary to the balloon remaining overdistended in a small peripheral vessel and rupturing.

Studies have shown that approximately 24% of Swan-Ganz catheters are malpositioned, as seen on an initial chest radiograph, and need to be repositioned.

Because of these potentially fatal consequences, it is imperative that a chest x-ray be obtained after insertion of a Swan-Ganz catheter.[47]

SENGTAKEN-BLAKEMORE TUBES

A specialized tube called a Sengstaken-Blakemore tube is used to temporarily occlude either esophageal or gastric veins in patients who enter the hospital with massive variceal bleeding. The tube has

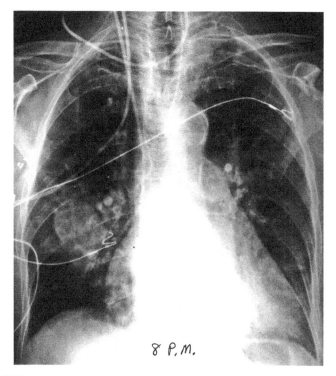

Figure 4.19 A repeat portable film at 8:00 P.M. after the catheter with-drawn, reveals a density representing an infarct or hemorrhage.

two balloons: A round distal balloon, which is inserted into the stomach, inflated, and pulled into the fundus of the stomach, that it is hoped will obliterate gastric varices (Figs 4.20 and 4.21). There is also an elliptical balloon that is inflated in the esophagus, which tamponades the esophageal varices.

There are numerous complications with Sengstaken-Blakemore tubes.

First and most serious is esophageal rupture, which occurs in approximately 15% of tube placements (Fig. 4.22).[48]

A chest film must be taken immediately after placing these tubes for further evaluation of potential complications, including esophageal perforation, aspiration pneumonia, and pneumothorax (Fig. 4.23).[49]

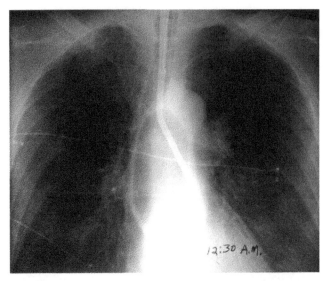

Figure 4.20 The proximal balloon on the Sengstaken-Blakemore tube is seen to be markedly inflated in the middle to distal esophagus.

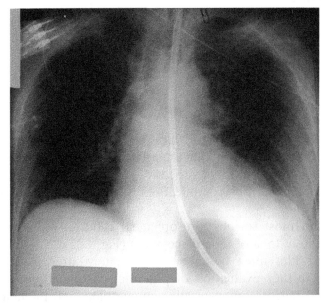

Figure 4.21 Distal balloon is in the fundus of the stomach.

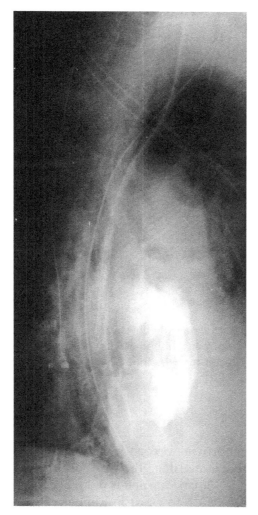

Figure 4.22   A lateral film taken after gastografin reveals a rupture of the esophagus, with contrast leaking into the posterior mediastinum.

INTRA-AORTIC BALLOON PUMPS

The intra-aortic balloon pump (IABP) is used to assist the left ventricle in patients with cardiogenic shock and left ventricular dysfunction.[50] This device is triggered by the ECG and a machine is used to inflate the balloon in diastole, which increases the pressure in the

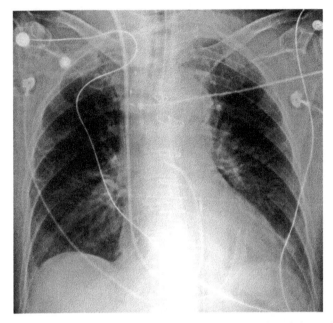

Figure 4.23 A Swan-Ganz catheter is seen entering the right pulmonary artery, and the endotracheal tube is in good position. An intra-aortic balloon pump has been inserted, but it is in poor position in the middle descending aorta.

proximal aorta, improving coronary blood flow. During systole, the balloon is deflated, diminishing the work of the left ventricle.

The balloon is 20–30 cm long and is radiolucent except for a radio-opaque marker at its tip to assist in radiographic localization. The tip should be just within the proximal descending thoracic aorta, distal to the origin of the main branches of the aortic arch and just distal to the origin of the left subclavian artery. A proximal location of the device results in cerebral and left upper extremity ischemia, and a distal location can occlude the mesenteric and renal vessels.[51] If the balloon is located too far inferiorly in the aorta, the pump may not function appropriately to increase coronary profusion and thus not decrease cardiac afterload. Another possible complication of an IABP is aortic dissection, which generally begins in the aorta just distal to the left subclavian artery.[52]

PACERS AND DEFIBRILLATORS

Pacemakers are used to treat various arrhythmias of the heart and heart block. The usual transvenous pacemaker is placed via the sub-clavian vein, so that the distal tip lies within the right ventricle.

It may have both atrial and ventricular lead wires, and these are connected to a pulse generator usually placed subcutaneously, in a pocket in the anterior chest wall. The lead wires are thin radio-opaque lines with electrodes attached to their tips. Correct place-ment of the lead is in the floor of the right ventricle, generally beneath the trabeculae at the apex. This provides contact with the endocardium, and within a few days, fibrin strands cover the tip, fixing the electrode to the right ventricular wall (Fig. 4.24).

On the frontal radiograph, the tranvenous right ventricular elec-trode should project slightly to the left of the midline and toward the ventricular apex. A bipolar catheter has an additional electrode in the right atrium (Fig. 4.25). In patients who have biventricular pacers, the left ventricular lead needs to enter the right atrium and then course posteriorly, entering the coronary sinus, out into one of

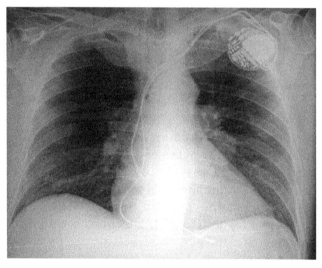

Figure 4.24   Note the excellent position of the bipolar pacer; one lead is embedded in the apex of the right ventricle and the other in the right atrium.

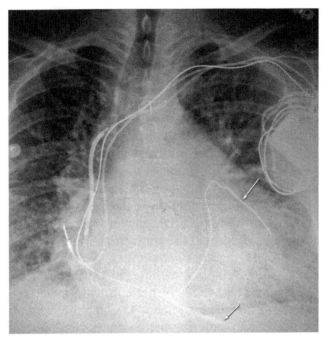

Figure 4.25 A patient with an enlarged heart and a bipolar pacer. The ventricular lead has the characteristic appearance of an intraventricular cardiac defibrillator. A pacemaker is seen in the right atrium, passing posteriorly through the coronary sinus and then out the veins on the posterior aspect of the left ventricle, permitting biventricular pacing.

the major veins that drain the left ventricle. A lateral film is necessary to follow the course of this lead.[53]

Malposition occurs in 3–14% of patients. Other complications seen include myocardial perforation, in which the tip of the transvenous pacemaker electrode can be seen projecting beyond the border of the heart. Unusual, but possible complications include hemopericardium or pericardial tamponade. Fracture of the wire is an infrequent complication but does occur in approximately 2% of patients. Pacemakers can be associated with infections, including soft tissue swelling, gas gangrene, and air–fluid levels at various sites, especially in the battery pocket.

Evaluate the battery site of a pacemaker. Loosening or infection can occur, and occasionally the patient will move and displace the

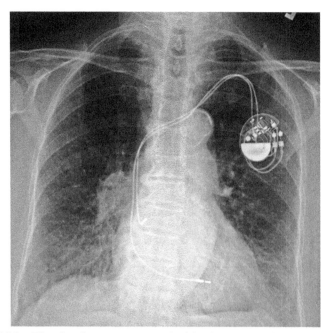

Figure 4.26   The classic appearance of a bipolar pacemaker reveals a pacer lead, placed distally into the trabecule of the right ventricle, and a right atrial lead.

battery, the so-called twiddlers syndrome. One must compare the present film with previous films, to see if there is a significant change in the insertion of the leads into the battery pack (Fig 4.26).[54]

Commonly, internal defibrillator devices are combined with a pacer. The internal defibrillator device is easily recognized on the chest radiograph by its characteristic configuration, with its tip lying in the right ventricle.

CHAPTER 5

BAROTRAUMA

Many patients in the ICU need mechanical ventilation, and *baro-trauma* refers to the potential consequences of this intervention. A significant number of ICU patients are intubated using either an endotracheal tube or a tracheotomy tube. Many patients receive positive end expiratory pressure (PEEP) ventilation.[55] Positive pressure ventilation (PPV) and PEEP ventilation greatly improve oxygenation in these patients and result in the opening of previously collapsed airways and alveoli. Of patients receiving PEEP, 5–15% have complications such as pneumothorax, mediastinal air, subcutaneous emphysema, or other extra alveolar air collections. Because many patients in the ICU have stiff lungs, the volume of a patient's lung can be increased by raising the base level of this pressure, called PEEP, in order to expand the lungs.[56] The effect of PEEP on blood oxygenation can be dramatic, due to the recruitment of alveoli initially not ventilated. It can, however, also overinflate ventilated alveoli. Be aware that the patient who has been placed on PEEP ventilation can have a radiograph that suggests he or she has improved dramatically, but this may be misleading simply because of the

ICU Chest Radiology: Principles and Case Studies, by Harold Moskowitz
Copyright © 2010 John Wiley & Sons, Inc.

increased air to tissue ratio, created artificially by the respirator. PEEP ventilation expands the lungs, making them more transparent and improving the patient's radiograph. Actually, radiologic changes are related only to the amount of air in the lung. The basic underlying process is still present; although the patient may look better on an x-ray, his or her clinical condition may be worse. Conversely, after a patient has been extubated or if the degree of PEEP ventilation is lowered, it may appear that a significant change has occurred. Due to loss of the overexpanded lung, the patient may look worse from a radiologic point of view but actually be better from a clinical view. Thus, when reading a radiograph to determine whether a patient has improved or gotten worse, it is important to know the level of PEEP ventilation and if the patient's positive pressure readings have changed. Only then can one make a judgment on a patient's status.[57]

PNEUMOTHORAX

Air within the pleural cavity, the potential space between the visceral and parietal pleura, is a *pneumothorax* (PTX). Pneumothorax can be caused either by a disruption of the visceral pleura, leading to air leaking from the lung outward, or sometimes by a disruption of the parietal pleura, in which atmospheric air is drawn inward, generally due to major trauma. PTX is rather commonly seen in the ICU secondarily to various procedures, especially thoracentesis, and it is the most frequently recognized form of extra-alveolar air in patients on ventilators (Fig. 5.1).[58]

Cardiac catheterization can also be a relatively common cause of pneumothorax; its incidence after subclavian vein puncture is between 0.3% and 3%, but it almost never occurs after internal jugular puncture.

Air outside the alveolus may have little clinical significance or may be a potentially life-threatening situation requiring immediate intervention. One must recognize air outside the alveolus, decide which anatomic compartment it is in, and (it is hoped) determine its cause.

Air accumulates in the least dependent portion of the hemithorax.[59] With the patient in the supine position, recognition of a pneumothorax is often difficult.[60] Air collects in the anterior inferior aspect of the thorax adjacent to the diaphragm. This produces a deep

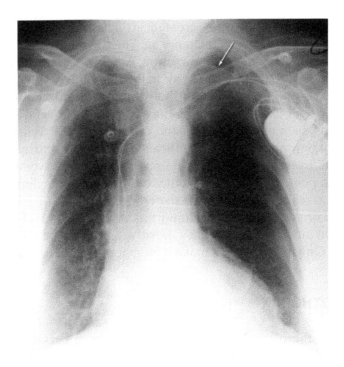

Figure 5.1 A hyperaerated patient with chronic cough and chest pain has a left-sided pneumothorax without a significant shift.

sulcus sign, an abnormal lucency replacing the diaphragmatic sulcus with air over the upper quadrant of the abdomen (Fig. 5.2).[61]

Detection of a pneumothorax is generally simple; one simply looks for the thin line of the visceral pleura. Other findings, however, may mimic a pneumothorax. Lines and tubes projecting over the lung can be confused with the visceral pleural surface. Skinfolds are a common problem, mimicking a pleural line and suggesting a pneumothorax. A gradual increase in opacity up to the questionable pneumothorax line is quite characteristic of a skinfold, and often one can follow skinfolds outside the thorax, thereby excluding the diagnosis. Pulmonary vessels peripheral to the visceral line can ensure that you are not dealing with a pneumothorax.[62]

A small pneumothorax can be seen on an upright film and is often missed on a supine film. Whenever a pneumothorax is suspected, an upright expiratory chest x-ray should be obtained.[63] Otherwise a cross-table lateral or decubitus view may be helpful. The decubitus

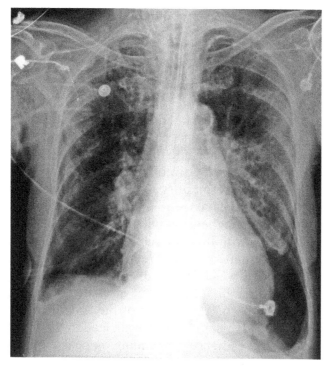

Figure 5.2 A patient with respiratory failure and chronic obstructive pulmonary disease has developed right-sided chest pain. Note the classic appearance of a deep sulcus sign on the left.

view, with the side of interest being highest and nondependent, is perhaps the most helpful in detecting a small pneumothorax. This view may even be superior to the erect view because it permits a higher degree of contrast between the air collection, the hemidiaphragm, and the lateral aspect of the ribs. Here also, careful attention must be paid to entities that may mimic pneumothorax, such as skinfolds, bandages, and other artifacts. Of course if there is a doubt, CT is excellent in demonstrating a pneumothorax, especially in emergency conditions, but getting an ICU patient to the CT room is always a difficult undertaking.

The characteristic radiologic features of a pneumothorax include the presence of a thin, opaque linear structure, beyond which there is an absence of vascular markings. This structure is the visceral pleura bordered on one side by air in the lung and on the other side by the air in the pleural cavity.

Mechanical ventilation can produce adverse effects, generally due to the overinflation of the alveoli, subsequent rupture, and escape of air into the interstitial septa.[64]

Most ventilator-induced barotrauma begins with interstitial pulmonary emphysema, which occurs when the intraalveolar pressure of the alveolus exceeds the pressure of the adjacent interstitium, permitting air to dissect into the interstitial tissues from the alveoli (Fig. 5.3).[65] Radiologically, one can occasionally see radiolucent streaks radiating from the hila into the peripheral lung. It is extremely important to recognize extra-alveolar air, which can lead to either sudden or progressive respiratory and cardiovascular collapse. In mechanically ventilated patients, a simple pneumothorax can rapidly become a life-threatening tension pneumothorax.[66]

PEEP also carries with it the possibility of severe adverse cardiopulmonary effects. There is often a reduction in cardiac blood flow due to PEEP or PPV, which is thought to be due to several factors, including an increase in intrathoracic pressure, which results in decreased venous return.[67] Distention of the alveoli can also cause compression of the alveolar capillary wall, leading to an increase in pulmonary vascular resistance. Depending on peak expiratory pressure and the duration of its use, PPV can also cause pulmonary edema and damage to the lung itself.[68]

Pneumothorax is the most frequently recognized manifestation of extra-alveolar air in patients who are on ventilator support. Subpleural blebs arise from air in peripheral interstitial tissues. These blebs enlarge and eventually rupture into the pleural space, causing a pneumothorax.[69] Mechanical ventilation may potentially increase the size of the pneumothorax rapidly, which can then lead to serious complications, such as tension pneumothorax and a significant shift of the mediastinum.[70] Recognize, however, that PEEP is often necessary to ventilate stiff lungs due to pneumonia, acute respiratory distress syndrome (ARDS), and/or pulmonary edema. In some patients, there may be pleural adhesions present, resulting in little or no shift of the mediastinum, even when there is significant tension. The incidence of pneumothorax in patients on mechanical ventilation has been reported at times to be as high as 25%.[71]

The radiologic signs of a massive pleural air collection include flattening of the cardiac border, shift of the mediastinum, and depression of the diaphragm. The radiologic diagnosis of a small

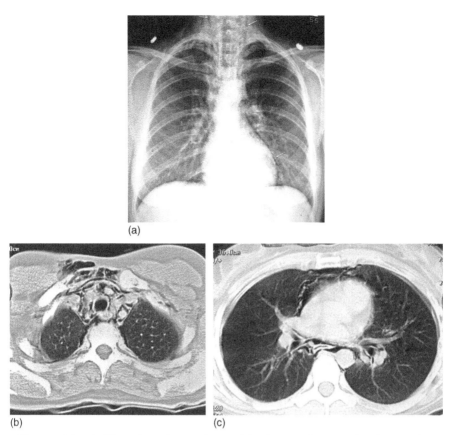

(a)

(b)   (c)

Figure 5.3 **A** The film of a patient with chest pain reveals air tracking along the mediastinum up into the neck and along the left cardiac border. This is the classic appearance of mediastinal emphysema. **B** A CT study of this patient's neck reveals the classic appearance of interstitial and mediastinal air tracking up into the neck and then into the soft tissues, anteriorly of the neck. **C** Another CT study reveals the classic appearance of air dissecting back into the mediastinum and the interstitial tissues of the chest. A small pneumothorax is seen anteriorly in the least dependent portion of the chest.

pneumothorax may not be easy because air tends to generally collect anteriorly in the anterior costophrenic sulcus. This is the highest portion of the thorax in supine patients. Air also collects in the subpulmonic recess. That explains the basilar lucencies, which, when seen, make the diaphragm, heart profiles, and anterior costrophrenic sulcus easily recognizable. Always remember that preexisting adhesions may cause a pneumothorax to remain encapsulated in one area even when the patient is erect.

PNEUMOMEDIASTINUM

The mediastinum is the central compartment of the thoracic cavity, located between the lungs and surrounded on all sides by parietal pleura. It extends from the sternum anteriorly to the vertebrae posteriorly, and contains the thymus, trachea, heart, great vessels, major bronchi, thoracic aorta, and the esophagus. Only two of the structures within the mediastinum can normally be air filled: the esophagus and, of course, the trachea. Air found in any other location within the mediastinum is pathologic and is referred to as pneumomediastinum.[72] This condition can be caused by esophageal rupture, tracheobronchial injuries, or alveolar rupture with retrograde flow of air into the mediastinum. Both esophageal and tracheal injuries require immediate intervention, whereas spontaneous pneumomediastinum can be watched, as it often does not have significant implications.

In a patient who has a pneumomediastinum, the radiograph will demonstrate well-defined lucencies around the heart and mediastinum. Extension of interstitial air can result in air in the soft tissue planes of the neck or even into the retroperitoneum.[73]

Air can also create a lucent stripe between the lung base and the central portion of the diaphragm so that it actually underlines the diaphramic portion of the heart. This often extends across the midline, giving rise to the continuous diaphragm sign.[74] Another radiologic finding occasionally seen is a lucent halo around the heart.

The shift of the mediastinal pleura away from the cardiac silhouette is yet another radiologic finding of pneumomediastinum. This membrane is seen as a linear, opaque structure that is outlined on both sides by air most commonly seen in the region of the aortopulmonary window.

Pneumomediastinum is best detected on a chest x-ray when air outlines the edge of an anatomic structure not normally visible, like the superior vena cava, left subclavian artery, left common carotid artery, or the right innominate artery.

TENSION PNEUMOTHORAX

A tension pneumothorax occurs when the pressure within the pleural space exceeds that of atmospheric pressure. The usual pathophysiology involves a valve-like mechanism in the lung, which, due to the normal negative-pressure breathing system opens upon inspiration, allowing air to flow into the pleural space, and closes upon expiration, thereby trapping the air. As air continues to enter the pleural space, the pressure within the pleura increases dramatically, forcing the mediastinum in the opposite direction. This shift of the mediastinum to the contralateral side results in a tension pneumothorax (Fig. 5.4).[75]

Tension PTX is a serious finding and must be treated via immediate insertion of a chest tube, as compression of the mediastinum

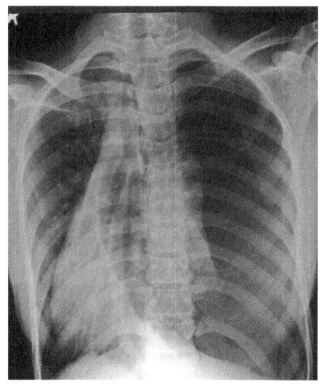

Figure 5.4   A classic example of tension pneumothorax, with a shift of the heart and mediastinium to the left.

compromises venous return to the heart. Death can be one of the consequences of this entity, if it is not immediately identified and corrected.

A most unusual manifestation of extra-alveolar air is air within the pericardium, known as pneumopericardium.[76] This condition is most often related to and caused by trauma, surgery, and/or infection. The radiologic findings include a lucent halo around the heart. On the upright radiograph, this lucency will continue only up to the level just above the main pulmonary artery. This condition is often mistaken for pneumomediastinum on a supine radiograph. It is important to remember that the pericardium ends at the vascular pedicle, so air seen superior to this point represents a pneumomediastinum. Remember, too, that both pneumopericardium and pneumomediastinum can occur together.

INTERSTITIAL EMPHYSEMA

Interstitial emphysema, a type of extra-alveolar air, occurs when pressure in the air spaces exceeds that within adjacent perivascular connective tissue and interlobular septa. When the alveolar-interstitial pressure exceeds a certain point, the alveoli immediately adjacent to the septa and connective tissue rupture, permitting air to enter the interstitium, leading to what is known as interstitial emphysema.[77] Air continues to dissect along a path of least resistance within the bronchovascular bundle, toward the hilum and/or the pleural surface. Further, air may travel into the mediastinum, leading to pneumomediastinum, or into the visceral pleura and pleural space, leading to pneumothorax (Fig. 5.5).

Interstitial emphysema can have a significant impact on cardiopulmonary function. For example, as the volume of air in the perivascular connective tissues of the lung increases, the pulmonary venous vessels collapse, causing increasing vascular resistance and subsequent shunting. In terms of oxygenation of the patient, especially in the patient with compromised pulmonary function, a decrease in lung volume secondary to interstitial air present can be detrimental.

Interstitial emphysema is not commonly appreciated in normally aerated lungs, because interstitial air is difficult to distinguish from intra-alveolar air. Also, a significant amount of alveolar consolidation is necessary to visualize this condition in its early

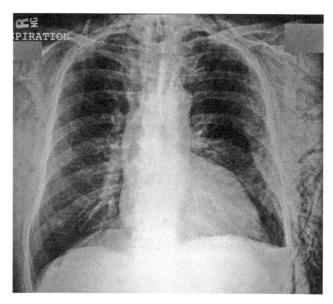

Figure 5.5   A portable film of a patient who had been in an automobile accident reveals rib fractures, a pneumothorax, and air in the mediastinum which has dissected into the chest wall, producing the characteristic of appearance of subcutaneous emphysema.

phase, until, eventually, large air cysts form, making visualization easier. The usual radiologic findings include fine linear or bubbly radiolucencies, often with an oval appearance, in a distribution that is patchy and nonconforming to the normal anatomic boundaries of the bronchopulmonary segments. These radiolucencies are often described as mottled. Streaky radiolucencies extending out from the hila to the periphery of the lung can also be seen.[78]

SUBCUTANEOUS EMPHYSEMA

Subcutaneous emphysema is a common finding in the ICU and is secondary to an air leak from a pneumothorax or a pneumomediastinum or following surgical procedures, such as the insertion of a chest tube (Fig. 5.6).[79]

Multiple configurations and lucencies are seen in the soft tissues. Often the air can dissect into muscle bundles and fascial planes up into the head and down into the abdomen, producing a characteristic radiologic configuration (Fig. 5.7).

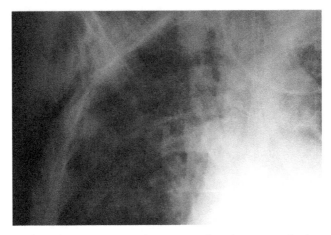

Figure 5.6 Interstitial air dissecting out to the pleura, producing pneumo-thorax and subcutaneous emphysema.

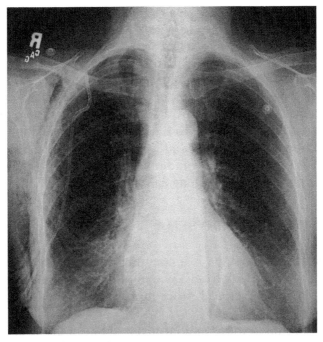

Figure 5.7 After the insertion of a chest tube, a small pneumothorax remains, and there is subcutaneous emphysema.

CHAPTER 6

PNEUMONIA

In the ICU, one of the most common causes of airspace disease is pneumonia, and yet it is often difficult to diagnose.[80] If there is a proper clinical story, such as the patient having fever, leukocytosis, and a new area of pulmonary infiltrate, the diagnosis of pneumonia can be made with relative certainty. This is not the usual scenario, since many cases of pneumonia in ICU patients are so called nosocomial.[81] This refers to a pneumonia that has been acquired while the patient has been a patient in the hospital. Pneumonias result in increased length of hospitalization which has a significant effect on mortality rates in ICU patients (Fig. 6.1).

The common pathogens in nosocomial pneumonia are aerobic gram negative organisms and *Staphylococcus aureus*.[82] Gram negative pneumonias have become much more frequent over the past two decades due to an older patient population and more medically diverse, and sicker, patients. The gram negative organisms are predominately *Pseudomonas aeruginosa, Klebsiella, Enterobacter*, and occasionally *Serratia*. These organisms are generally present in the ICU, and oropharyngeal colonization occurs rapidly.

ICU Chest Radiology: Principles and Case Studies, by Harold Moskowitz
Copyright © 2010 John Wiley & Sons, Inc.

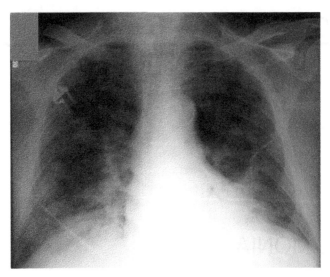

Figure 6.1   A patient in the ICU who had been intubated for almost a week developed classic bilateral lower lobe pneumonia, probably secondary to aspiration. This is the classic presentation of nosocomial pneumonia.

A patient admitted to a medical ICU rapidly becomes infected with gram negative organisms. Oropharyngeal colonization sets the stage for aspiration into the trachea and lower lung fields, leading to the development of pneumonia.[83] The majority of gram negative pneumonias in the ICU are due to prior oropharyngeal colonization.[84] In some hospitals, *Staphylococcus aureus* remains a major nosocomial etiologic agent, due to the development of methicillin resistant strains. Unusual agents such as *Legionella*[85] have been responsible for several outbreaks of pneumonia, especially in elderly patients, secondary to contaminated hospital water sources. Immunocompromised patients and patients who have been on steroids or immunosuppressant drugs may develop unusual infections with organisms such as *Aspergillus* or mucormycosis.[86]

Diabetes is an additional risk factor, and on occasion we see a diabetic patient with *Candida* pneumonia.[87]

The risk of a patient developing a nosocomial infection is 10–25% higher in patients who require intubation and mechanical ventilation than in other patients.[88] The endotracheal tube or tracheostomy tube allows the direct access of bacteria to the lower respiratory tract. The mechanical trauma to the tracheal wall may predispose the patient to the development of pneumonia.

Both the pharynx and the stomach are reservoirs for gram negative organisms, which are the precursors of the development of pneumonia in intubated patients. About 25% of patients who are intubated for more than 3–4 days will develop pneumonia.[89] Another abnormality to search for on the chest radiograph is an air–fluid level above the lucency of a cuffed endotracheal tube. This represents fluid caught in the pharynx above the balloon; if present, this should be suctioned regularly to prevent aspiration.[90]

There is often retrograde colonization of the pharynx and the trachea from the stomach. This may also occur secondary to nasogastric tube placement. The tube may interfere with the lower esophageal sphincter, increasing the incidence of reflux and, eventually, tracheal involvement. Feeding the patient via tube in order to meet increased caloric needs also leads to a higher incidence of reflux and the development of pneumonia. In an effort to decrease the incidence of reflux, one may occasionally consider the possibility of feeding the patient via a jejunal tube. Most studies show that the predominant factor in the development of nosocomial pneumonia is aspiration of pharyngeal or gastric fluid in the mechanically ventilated patient.[91] We must not forget, however, that approximately 25% of all pneumonias may be due to a primary pneumonia or a pneumonia secondary to a blood-borne infection. Respiratory therapy equipment may also be a potential source of bacterial contamination and subsequent pneumonia, and one must not forget that the hands of the health worker, which pass from patient to patient, are colonized with various types of bacteria and are a potential source of contamination among patients.[92]

A diagnosis of a nosocomial pneumonia may be reliably straightforward when the clinical picture reveals an intubated patient who has developed fever and leucocytosis while in the ICU. But in the ICU patient, many of whom have many other sources of pulmonary infiltrates, the diagnosis of pneumonia is not so evident. People have attempted to make the diagnosis via invasive methods such as transtracheal or fiberoptic broncoscopy. These techniques have never been shown to improve outcome or survival, and their utility is questionable.

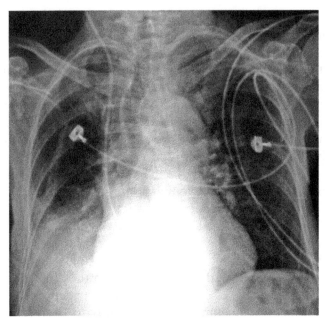

Figure 6.2 A portable film reveals a classic silhouette sign. Note the obliteration of the right hemidiaphragm with preservation of the right cardiac border, indicating there is pneumonia in the right lower lobe, although the right middle lobe still aerating well.

The radiologic evaluation reveals confluent opacities with ill-defined borders and, occasionally, loss of the cardiac or diaphragmatic border, the silhouette sign (Fig. 6.2).

Air bronchograms are often seen and are helpful in establishing the diagnosis (Fig. 6.3).

Occasionally, in a patient with a new air space opacity, the diagnosis may be simple. However, in patients who have either atelectasis, hemorrhage, pulmonary infarcts, pulmonary contusions, pulmonary edema, or ARDS, this diagnosis is not easy to make because multiple conditions often co-exist.[93] Many of these pulmonary opacities simulate pneumonia; however, on autopsy, other entities clearly represent a sizable percentage of abnormalities seen in these patients.[94]

One of the more useful signs indicating a nosocomial infection is an air space process abutting a fissure. Air bronchograms are also highly suggestive, and the silhouette sign, obliteration of the diaphragmatic or cardiac surface, can be helpful.

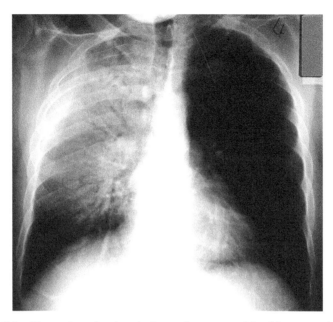

Figure 6.3 Note the classic air bronchogram with this extensive right upper lobe pneumonia.

Gram negative bacteria and *Staphylococcus aureus* are well known causes of cavitary pneumonia. Thus cavitation is a sign that should suggest nosocomial infection.

Basilar atelectasis, without signs of volume loss, is often misinterpreted as pneumonia. Rapid changes in a pulmonary opacity indicate probable atelectasis, especially in the lower lobes (Fig. 6.4).

The possibility of aspiration pneumonia, especially in patients with lower lobe opacities, should always be a consideration. The distribution of the abnormality reflects patient position at the time of the aspiration. The basal segments of the right lower lobe are those most commonly involved in patients who are erect. In supine patients, especially in those who are ill, the posterior basal segments or the superior segments of the lower lobes are the most dependent segments and, most often, the site of aspiration pneumonia. Occasionally, these areas may be seen as a round area, the so-called round pneumonia (Fig. 6.5).[95]

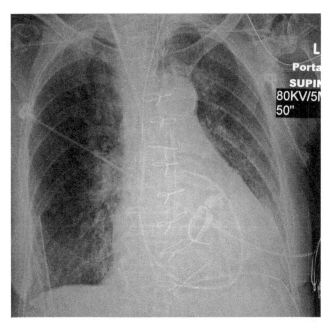

Figure 6.4 After mitral valve replacement surgery, the patient has obliteration of left hemidiaphragm and density behind the heart due to left lower lobe pneumonia.

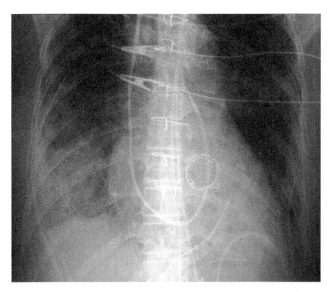

Figure 6.5 After mitral valve replacement surgery, the patient has developed an infiltrate in a peculiar round configuration, representing a round pneumonia.

Pneumonias can be classified as either lobar, bronchopneumonia, or interstitial (Fig. 6.6). A lobar infection can be thought of as a consolidation, filling the entire lobe of a lung with fluid. This is often due to streptococcus infection. The typical radiographic appearance is a homogenous consolidation, filling an entire lobe all the way to the pleura. An air bronchogram is almost always present.

Occasionally, other organisms causing pneumonia produce findings that suggest their etiology—for example, *Klebsiella pneumonia*, a gram negative necrotizing bacteria, causes the lobe to expand in a characteristic way, producing bulging of the fissures (Figs. 6.7 and 6.8).

Other gram negative bacteria, such as *Pseudomonas*, can cause consolidation with cavity formation.[96]

Bronchopneumonia probably starts as the peribronchial focus of infection that spreads to the alveoli. It appears on the x-ray as a patchy, fluffy opacity that will often go on to coalesce. The acute infection fills both the bronchus and the alveolus, so an air bronchogram is seldom visible, and there is usually no volume

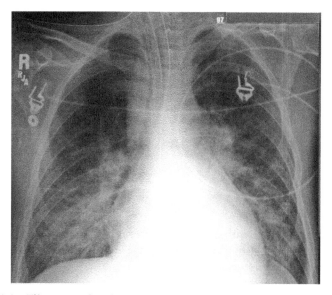

Figure 6.6   Film of an intubated patient reveals bilateral infiltrates. These lower lobe pneumonias can simulate areas of atelectasis.

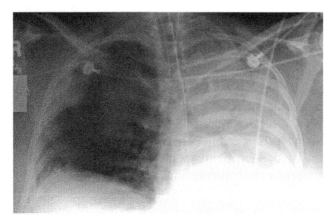

Figure 6.7 A patient with extensive left-sided pneumonia, which has caused consolidation of the entire lung with a shift of the mediastinum to the left. Note the beautiful air bronchogram, left pneumonia, and shift of the mediastinum.

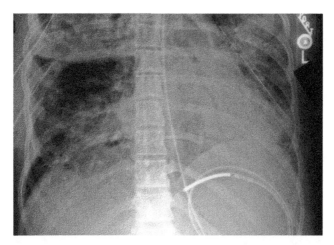

Figure 6.8 A patient with extensive bilateral pneumonia. The right upper lobe is consolidated with a downward bulge of the horizontal fissure. This patient has *Klepsiella pneumonia.*

loss. The common organisms producing bronchopneumonia are staphylococci, but other bacteria such as gram negative aerobes and other anaerobes may be implicated.

Interstitial pneumonias in the ICU are rare but often can extend and involve the acini of the lung. An extensive interstitial process can simulate an alveolar process due to overlapping densities. While uncommon, interstitial pneumonia is often due to viral organisms, such as microplasma pneumonia.

Remember that in a patient with AIDS, the usual pneumonias encountered are initially interstitial or occasionally, nodular, which then become alveolar.[97]

Pneumoncystis carinii pneumonia typically presents with a fine interstitial process that often goes on to alveolar consolidation. Cytomegalovirus (CMV) is another frequent cause of interstitial infiltrates and is frequent in AIDS patients, although many cases are not diagnosed until an autopsy has been performed. Fungal diseases such as histoplasmosis[98] or tuberculosis often present with nodular lesions and must be distinguished from other nodular lesions, such as metastatic tumors or the occasional lymphoma.

The chest x-ray underestimates the presence of pneumonia (Fig. 6.9).

A CT examination is much more sensitive than the usual AP film (Fig. 6.10). Studies suggest that the portable film fails to demonstrate

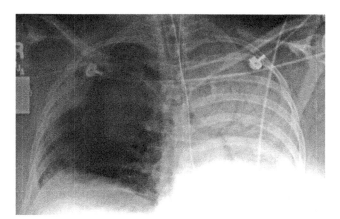

Figure 6.9 Extensive pneumonia in entire left lung. Questionable right peripheral pneumonia.

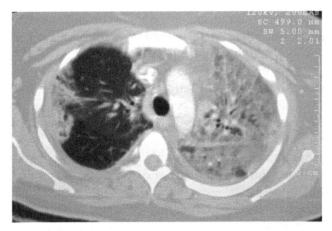

Figure 6.10   A CT scan reveals extensive pneumonia throughout the left lung, with small areas of pneumatocels. Note the extensive right-sided pneumonia, which was barely visible on the plain film, probably secondary to *Pneumocystics carinii* pneumonia in a patient with AIDS.

basilar lung consolidation in 26% of patients. It is important to adequately visualize the retrocardiac and retrodiaphragmatic areas; the use of grids when obtaining a portable chest x-ray significantly improves visualization of these areas.

CT, being highly sensitive for detecting lung abnormalities due to its improved contrast resolution, permits us to better evaluate a chest abnormality and to make certain inferences. Atelectasis reveals displacement of the fissures and crowding of the vessels and bronchi. Often the amount of fluid seen on the chest CT is considerable, more than was expected on a review of a simple portable film. The characteristic appearance of a pulmonary infarct is also better seen on a CT study.

NODULAR IN FILTRATES

Most often, multiple pulmonary nodules represent metastatic deposits throughout the lung. However, in the ICU population, occasionally multiple nodules can have different etiologies. We often see septic emboli either from injection by an IV drug abuser or from a

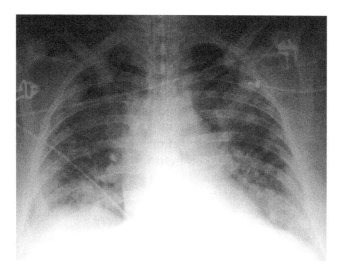

Figure 6.11   A patient with an infected tricuspid valve and septic emboli throughout both lung fields.

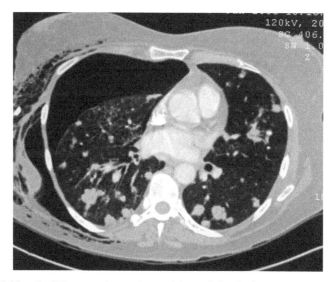

Figure 6.12   A CT scan of a patient with nodular lesions reveals the classic appearance of metastatic disease. Note the sharp configuration to the nodules, which is quite different from those secondary to infected emboli. Also seen is a large pneumonthorax and subcutaneous emphysema.

patient who has infected tricuspid endocarditis.[99] This may produce multiple nodules throughout both lung fields (Fig. 6.11).

In the immunocompromised patient, there are many diagnostic possibilities; the most common fungi are *Aspergillus, Cryptococcus*, tuberculosis, and possibly histoplasmosis. In a patient who has had a transplant, the possibility of lymphoprolypherative disorders may present as nodules.[100] Remember, in a patient with multiple nodules, but even in a patient with a solitary mass or a solitary nodule, one should look for films taken before the patient came to the ICU (Fig. 6.12).

Understanding the course and growth of a nodule or determining its density in the ICU patient is extremely helpful in arriving at a correct diagnosis.

CHAPTER 7

PULMONARY EDEMA

Many patients either have pulmonary edema on admission to the ICU or develop it while a patient in the ICU. Pulmonary edema results in decreased capillary oxygenation. There are many and varied etiologies that cause pulmonary edema. It can be classified as either hydrostatic or due to increased permeability.[101] In spite of the differences in etiology, the common denominator is an overabundance of water in the extravascular space. Treatment is best when individually tailored to the specific cause of a particular patient's pulmonary edema, and often that etiology can be suspected from a careful understanding of the abnormalities seen on the portable chest radiograph.[102]

In normal conditions, there is movement of fluids between the intravascular and the extravascular spaces at the alveolar capillary level. Water moves out on the pulmonary arterial side due to the difference in hydrostatic pressure, and this fluid moves back into the capillary from the venous side as a result of oncotic pressure. In normal conditions, there is a balance between the hydrostatic and

ICU Chest Radiology: Principles and Case Studies, by Harold Moskowitz
Copyright © 2010 John Wiley & Sons, Inc.

the oncotic pressures, which occurs only if there is an intact membrane at the alveolocapillary level.[103]

Another important feature to remember is the normal anatomy of the lung. Basically, the air space consists of a normal alveolus and the interstitium. The interstitium consists of the wall of the alveolus, the bronchus, and the tissue surrounding the vessels. The alveolus consists of type I and type II pneumocytes overlying a basement membrane.

As the left ventricle begins to fail, there is an increase in the left ventricular end diastolic pressure. This results in increased pressure in the left atrium, and then increased pressure back into the pulmonary venous system. This is referred to as pulmonary venous hypertension and can be measured when a Swan-Ganz catheter is wedged and measures the pulmonary capillary wedge pressure.[104] This rise in the pulmonary capillary wedge pressure indicates an increase in extravascular water in the lungs, eventually producing extra volume in the interstitium and then, eventually, in the alveoli. This is called hydrostatic pulmonary edema, also known as cardiogenic pulmonary edema, which produces a classic appearance on the x-ray.[105] Hydrostatic pulmonary edema can also be due to overhydration of a patient and, occasionally, renal failure.

Another form of pulmonary edema is noncardiac pulmonary edema, which occurs due to an increase in the capillary permeability.[106] There are many etiologies for this, including pneumonia, trauma, and aspiration as well as extra pulmonary causes, such as sepsis, shock, neurogenic pulmonary edema, and drug toxicity. In this entity, the capillary membrane becomes more permeable to fluids moving from the vascular compartment directly into the alveoli, to produce a so-called permeability or injury edema. In this situation, cardiac function can be normal. It is important to remember that cardiogenic pulmonary edema and noncardicgenic pulmonary edema can be present in a patient at the same time. Cardiac pulmonary edema is most commonly due to left ventricular failure of any origin, whereas noncardic pulmonary edema is generally seen in ARDS.[107]

There are various methods of distinguishing among the multiple etiologies of pulmonary edema. Invasive methods, such as pulmonary artery pressure measurements (Swan-Ganz catheter), are often used. The portable chest radiograph, however, is the most commonly used noninvasive study to identify the presence of pulmonary edema

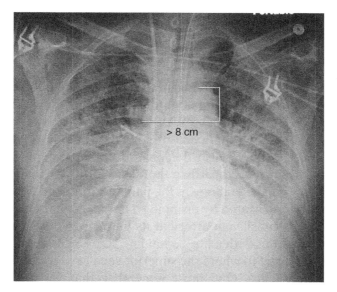

Figure 7.1   A patient in failure with bilateral pulmonary edema and a widened vascular pedicle, >8 cm.

in the ICU patient.[108] The chest radiograph offers clues to the cause of the patient's fluid overload. Cardiogenic pulmonary edema involves failure of the cardiac pump and can be due to either myocardial or valvular disease.

The classic findings of congestive heart failure depend on the severity of the failure of the left ventricle. The upright chest x-ray is more accurate than the supine portable film in depicting these findings (Fig. 7.1). The earliest sign of pulmonary edema is vascular redistribution, or so-called cephalization, and this is the earliest sign of pulmonary venous hypertension. As the ventricle continues to fail, perivascular and peribronchial cuffing occurs, and eventually interstitial and intralobular septal thickening is seen. This thickening is seen on the x-ray as straight, short linear lines at the edges of the lung called Kerley B lines. Pleural effusions may occur, and as the intravascular hydrostatic pressure continues to rise, fluid begins to fill the air spaces, resulting in alveolar edema. Aveolar edema classically produces air space consolidation in the middle to upper lung fields, but it can also involve the lower lung fields especially in patients who have COPD.[109] This situation can mimic pneumonia radiographically, and one should be careful to make this distinction. In patients who have pulmonary edema, treatment of the edema will rapidly cause these areas of alveolar edema to disappear. Pneumonia takes much longer to resolve.

Milne and colleagues[110] demonstrated that one can obtain a large amount of useful hemodynamic information from consideration of the vascular pedicle width (VPW).

VPW is often important in determining the etiology of pulmonary edema. Milne's group[111] also demonstrated that using VPW combined with the increased cardiac thoracic ratio is the most helpful sign in elucidating the etiology of the patient's problem. The vascular pedicle width is measured by dropping a perpendicular line from the edge of the left subclavian artery at its junction with the aorta and then connecting this with a horizontal line across the cardiac shadow to a point just distal to where the superior vena cava crosses the right main stem bronchus. One must remember that vascular pedicle width gives us an estimation of intravascular volume status. This width should be 7–8 cm. The cardiothoracic ratio is evaluated by dividing the widest transverse diameter of the cardiac silhouette by the widest transverse diameter of the thorax, just above the diaphragm. Anything above 50% represents cardiomegaly.

Normally there is a balance between the capillary pressure and the plasma oncotic pressure, so the alveolus remains free of fluid. (The plasma oncotic pressure is the pressure exerted by the proteins.) The integrity of the capillary wall is important in maintaining this normal homeostatic mechanism. Damage to the membrane allows fluid and proteins to enter the interstitium of the lung, thus changing pressure relationships. The lymphatics of the lung play a critical role in eliminating fluid from the interstitum, and they can be discerned on the chest radiograph when filled with fluid. Normally, the flow across the capillary membrane is determined by the Starling equation. From the interstitium of the lung, fluids and proteins are picked up by the lymphatic system and brought back into the bloodstream. The capillary pressure drives fluids across the capillary membrane into the interstitium when this pressure exceeds 8 mm Hg. The plasma colloid osmotic pressure causes fluids to move back from the interstitium into the pulmonary capillary. Normal plasma oncotic pressure exerted by plasma proteins is approximately 25 mm Hg, ensuring a normal flow of water back out of the extravascular space

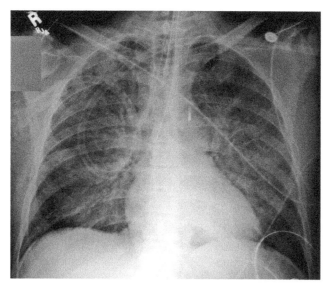

Figure 7.2   The film of a patient who was admitted with an acute myocardial infarction reveals the classic appearance of increased blood flow to the upper lobes, cephalization. Note the excellent position of the intraortic balloon pump just distal to the origin of the left subclavian artery.

into the capillaries. Pulmonary edema can result when either the hydrostatic pressure has increased or, occasionally, when the colloid osmotic pressure is markedly decreased. This decrease in plasma proteins has to be quite significant and so is a rare occurrence. On the other hand, pulmonary venous hypertension is the most common cause of pulmonary edema.

One can fairly adequately determine left ventricular end-diastolic pressure and thus the degree of failure demonstrated on the chest x-ray, if some simple basic principles are followed.[112] This often determines how to treat a patient. The first abnormality that occurs is a redistribution of blood to the upper lobe pulmonary veins, so-called cephalization (Fig. 7.2).

This occurs due to vasoconstriction in the lower lobes and occurs when left ventricular end-diastolic pressure reaches 10–14 mm Hg.

As the pressure in the left ventricle continues to increase, fluid begins to accumulate in the perivascular spaces. There is blurring of the sharpness of the vessels, as there is now fluid between the wall

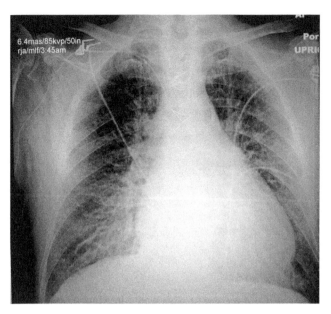

Figure 7.3   A patient with marked cardiomegaly and left ventricular endia-stolic pressure elevated to 15–16 mm Hg. Note the increased flow to the upper lobe veins as well the indistinct vascular markings secondary to peri-vascular cuffing.

of the vessels and the surrounding alveoli. This so-called perivascular cuffing occurs at a left ventricular end-diastolic pressure somewhere between 14 and 18 mm Hg (Fig. 7.3).

As the pressure continues to increase, there is transudation of fluid into the interstitium, first in the tissue surrounding the bronchi and then within the lymphatics. These lymphatics carry fluid away to the periphery of the lung. This results in an interstitial pattern in the lungs, called Kerley B lines, which can best be seen in the periphery of the lung abutting the pleural surface, at right angles to the pleural surface (Fig. 7.4).

This occurs at left ventricular end-diastolic pressure somewhere between 18 and 22 mm Hg. At this time, the patient is classically symptomatic, developing a wheeze due to the interstitial fluid within the lungs. This so-called cardiac asthma should not be mistaken for a routine patient with asthma, because their respective treatments are completely different.

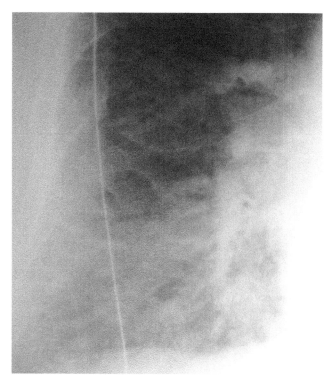

Figure 7.4   Note the classic appearance of linear lines perpendicular to the pleural surface, representing fluid in the lymphatics adjacent to the pleura, the so-called Kerley B lines.

As the pressure exceeds 25 mm Hg, fluid will accumulate in the alveolus itself, producing the classic pattern of pulmonary edema. Fluid can spread from alveolus to alveolus through the pores of Kohn. On the x-ray, the classic pattern of extensive alveolar fluid, the so-called bat or angel wings, will be seen (Fig. 7.5).

Remember to look for these characteristic signs: cardiac size, cephalization, peribronchial cuffing, septal lines, alveolar edema, and pleural effusions.[113]

Cardiac size, including the size of the left ventricle and the other cardiac chambers, is extremely important in accessing the etiology of pulmonary edema (Fig. 7.6). The size of the left ventricle can be estimated on the PA and lateral views. On the lateral view, if the left ventricular border extends beyond the inferior vena cava, it

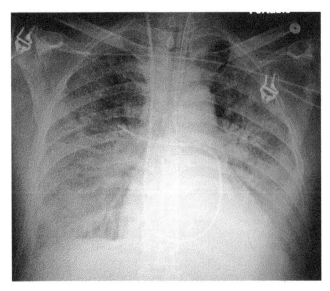

Figure 7.5   A patient in failure with classic perihilar alveolar edema, producing the characteristic angel or bat wing configuration.

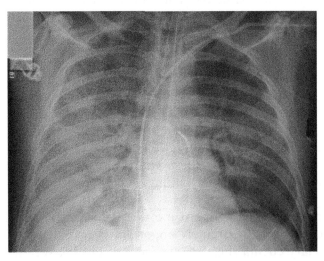

Figure 7.6   A patient in failure after an acute MI who lay on his right side, producing the typical appearance of unilateral pulmonary edema.

signifies left ventricular enlargement. Note also that the size of the left atrium can be estimated on the AP or PA film. If there is a convexity to the left border of the heart below the bulge of the pulmonary artery, the left auricle is enlarged, and thus the left atrium is significantly enlarged. In addition, the left atrium will elevate the left mainstem bronchus, producing an increase in the angle at the carina. Occasionally, as the left atrium enlarges, a density will be seen to the right of the vertebral column, the so called double-density sign of left atrial enlargement.[114]

The azygous vein is also a significant indicator of venous pressure. When it bows forward and enters into the superior vena cava just above the right upper lobe bronchus, it can be easily visualized and measured. The size of the azygous vein varies, although when it is significantly over 7–8 mm there is likely venous hypertension.

Although pulmonary edema is most often bilateral, it can occasionally be unilateral. This can be due to simple things, such as the patient lying on one side in the decubitus position or underlying disorders of the lung that result in differential blood flow.

Also, rapid reexpansion of the lung after treatment for a pneumothorax or atelectisis can cause reexpansion edema, which may present as unilateral edema.[115]

It is important to consider factors that alter the vascular pedicle width artificially, such as patient rotation, the supine position, inadequate inspiration, certain ventilator settings, and the patient's body habitus. It is important to take these factors into account when one evaluates the patient's volume status.

One must always remember that there are many factors that go into your evaluation of the chest x-ray. Underlying etiologies, such as chronic obstructive lung disease, pulmonary fibrosis, and co-existing pneumonias, may alter the appearance of the patient with pulmonary edema.[116] PEEP can affect the appearance of the chest x-ray, and although we attempt to obtain the film at the end of inspiration, this does not always occur in the ICU setting.

While the portable x-ray is often useful in distinguishing the various types of pulmonary edema, it is not always possible to distinguish cardiogenic and noncardiogenic causes. In general, congestive failure as the cause of edema includes a widened vascular pedicle, perivascular cuffing, septal thickening, and pleural effusions. The alveolar and air space capacities tend to be central and uniform.

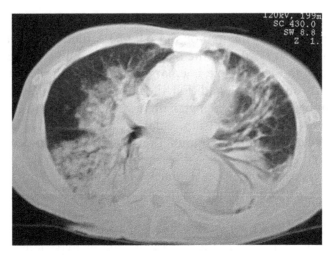

Figure 7.7   A CT study is more exquisitely sensitive in visualizing alveolar densities than is an x-ray film. Note the alveoli filled with fluid and the uniformity of the fluid in a patient with pulmonary edema.

A CT scan is much more sensitive for demonstrating these findings than is the portable chest x-ray (Fig. 7.7). One thing to keep in mind is the variable appearance that can occur as air space densities are clearing. They may clear from various areas of the lung at different rates and produce a patchy irregular appearance. Review of recent serial chest x-rays demonstrate this as rapidly changing air space densities, favoring the diagnosis of congestive heart failure over ARDS or pneumonia.

Another cause of pulmonary edema is overhydration. Often enthusiastic fluid replacement, especially in the operating room, results in pulmonary edema and third spacing of significant amounts of fluids. In the upright portable chest radiograph, cephalization is not seen secondary to overhydration. A balanced distribution of fluid is seen in overhydration, and there are new infiltrates. Overhydration increases the width of the vascular pedicle due to an increase in vascular volume.

Noncardiac pulmonary edema may be seen after near drowning, after acute head trauma, drug overdose, or inhalation injuries. These are uncommon causes of pulmonary edema, and the pathophysiology of this entity is often unclear. Most often the diagnosis is made in light of the clinical history rather than a specific x-ray edema pattern. Also remember that abnormalities in renal function and the presence of renal failure will result in an inability to excrete fluid, increasing the pulmonary vascular volume and causing significant amounts of fluid to accumulate in the body, which "third spaces."

Increased permeability pulmonary edema, or so-called leaky lung syndrome, is another form of noncardiogenic pulmonary edema.[117] Distinguishing hydrostatic from increased permeability pulmonary edema can be difficult. One distinguishing feature is that in noncardiogenic pulmonary edema there is often the appearance of patchy peripheral infiltrates. The vascular pedicle remains small or normal in size, and air bronchograms are common. Septal lines are uncommon. Various types of pneumonitis or hemorrhage can produce radiographic findings that may be indistinguishable. One must remember that the imaging findings can only supplement the information obtained from physical examination and clinical history, and all these three together are crucial in making a correct diagnosis. Leaky lung syndrome (LLS) is a form of noncardiogenic pulmonary edema that can be thought of as part of a continuum, with LLS a mild manifestation of acute lung injury and ARDS at the other end of the spectrum. The radiographic and CT findings of ARDS are described in the next chapter.

CHAPTER 8

ACUTE RESPIRATORY DISTRESS SYNDROME

Acute respiratory distress syndrome (ARDS) is a clinical syndrome representing an advanced form of increased permeability (noncardiogenic) pulmonary edema. Acute lung injury (ALI) has many etiologies, which result in a large spectrum of clinical presentations, ARDS is the most severe. The entity was first described, in 1967 by Ashbaugh et al.[118] in 1969, as a triad of pulmonary edema, congestion, and atelectasis. They reported that the edema was a result of increased capillary permeability, leading to an accumulation of a protein-rich exudative fluid in the alveolus. During the past 40 years it has become apparent that this disease has a spectrum, and there are many direct and indirect causes.

Many etiologies cause damage to the lung, including the inhalation of noxious stimuli like toxic fumes or gases, drowning, or aspiration of gastric contents (Mendelson syndrome). Vascular causes of ARDS result from fat embolism, toxins from sepsis, acute pancreatitis, or blood transfusions. While the etiologies differ, the clinical and radiologic findings are similar.[119] The diagnosis of ARDS is a clinical one, presenting with bilateral infiltrates consistent with

ICU Chest Radiology: Principles and Case Studies, by Harold Moskowitz
Copyright © 2010 John Wiley & Sons, Inc.

alveolar fluid, secondary to increased pulmonary vascular permeability. It is interesting that in spite of the sophisticated support available in the modern ICU, the mortality from this entity has not significantly improved over the past 20 years. Some of this is due to the increasingly older patients in today's ICU as well as to the increasing prevalence of sepsis and multiorgan failure. Whether the patients have multiorgan failure due to ARDS or whether the ARDS is secondary to the patients' organ failure is not clear.

The radiographic appearance of ARDS varies with the stage of the disease, and depends somewhat on the underlying lung abnormalities of the patient, the severity of the lung injury, and any associated complications such as secondary pneumonia, congestive heart failure, or barotrauma.[120]

For the first 24–72 h the chest x-ray usually does not show significant findings and lags behind the hypoxia that most patients experience.

The first radiographic abnormalities seen are bilateral patchy air space areas of consolidation (Fig. 8.1). This corresponds to the exudate phase of ARDS, when a large amount of protein-rich pul-

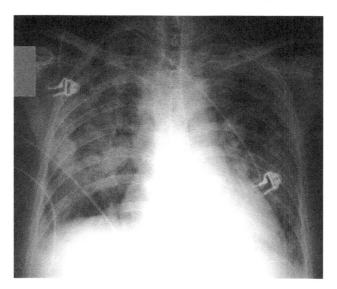

Figure 8.1   The film reveals patchy, fairly early confluent areas of infiltrate throughout both lung fields; the air bronchograms are difficult to visualize in the left lower lobe.

monary edema leaks into the alveoli. Soon there is proliferation of type II pneumocytes and the formation of a hyaline membrane (Fig. 8.2). Eventually, the individual patchy, scattered areas of opacity, which are quite diffuse, begin to coalesce, often with a lower lobe predominance (Fig. 8.3).[121]

Air bronchograms are commonly identified because the exudative process is very thick and involves the alveoli and the interstitium, but the fluid does not usually extend into the bronchi, which remain patent.

The findings may not change for days, possibly weeks, which is in sharp contrast to alveolar opacities secondary to cardiogenic edema or even pneumonia, which change more rapidly.[122]

Much remains to be understood about ARDS. One can consider it an imbalance between injury and repair, and the actual changes are quite complex. The specific site of injury is the alveolar capillary membrane, whose endothelium becomes permeable, permitting

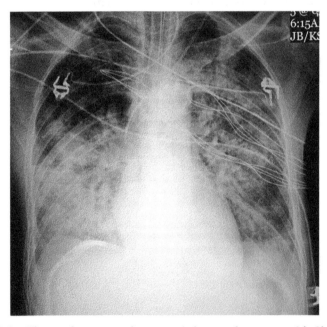

Figure 8.2 The coalescence of many of the patchy areas of infiltrate are seen throughout both lung fields, which eventually will create a more homogenous and extensive infiltrate.

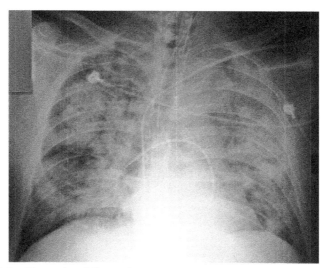

Figure 8.3 Extensive bilateral coalescent densities that have progressed over several days; note the classic air bronchograms.

transcapillary migration of proteinaceous fluid and inflammatory cells into the alveoli as well as the interstitium. The alveolar basement membrane sluffs, as part of the repair process, and a hyaline membrane forms, secondary to the migration of the protein-rich edema fluid. The type II pneumocyte has been denuded and gas exchange is impaired. The patient becomes markedly hypoxic, cyanotic, and dyspneic Oxygen saturation falls, necessitating increased levels of PEEP, to, it is hoped, recruit and open other alveoli (Fig. 8.4). The danger is that overdistention of normally air-filled alveoli results in secondary barotraumas, complicating the patient's ARDS.[123]

Also, superimposed pneumonia occurs frequently, which can be inferred by focal consolidation (or worsening of opacities) after a relatively stable phase. Sometimes CT may be necessary to evaluate a persistent source of sepsis, and one may see other abnormalities such as cavitating lesions.

CT plays a significant role in evaluating a patient with ARDS (Fig. 8.5). As stated earlier, this syndrome of acute lung injury proceeds from areas of ground glass opacity, which resolve fairly quickly, to severe ARDS with superimposed infections and possible barotrauma. All of these can be identified better on a CT scan, although

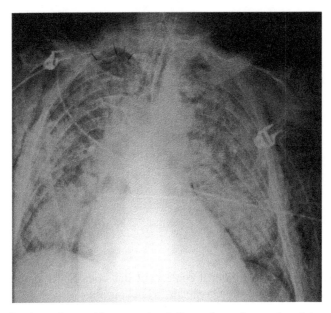

Figure 8.4   A patient with extensive bilateral confluent densities while on PEEP has developed a pneumothrax and subcutaneous emphysema on the right.

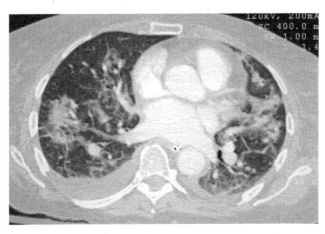

Figure 8.5   A CT study of a patient with bilateral confluent densities reveals the extensive alveolar component with early air bronchograms.

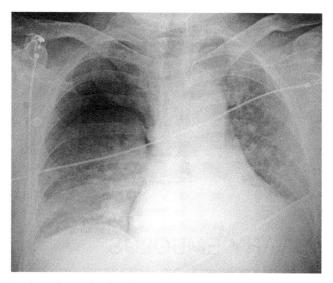

Figure 8.6   A patient who had just been extubated after 10 days of assisted ventilation developed marked shortness of breath. A large pneumothrax is seen.

bringing the sick patient to the scanner does provide logistical problems.[124] In ARDS, there are primarily extensive air-filled opacities, with air bronchograms within the consolidative areas.

Patchy areas of relatively normal appearing parenchyma are often present.[125] Often CT will demonstrate evidence of barotrauma such as pneumothorax, small pneumatocoeles, or air in the mediatinium (Fig. 8.6).

The recovery phase of ARDS occurs slowly, and often there is replacement of the consolidative opacities with vesicular and fibrotic changes.[126] Traction bronchieatasis is commonly seen as well as bronchiolectasis. Although many of these findings may slowly regress, fibrotic changes may persist with secondary architectural distortion. A lower diffusion capacity is commonly encountered, which persists. Many of the abnormal spirometic parameters revert to normal at the end of 6–12 months.

CHAPTER 9

PULMONARY EMBOLUS

Pulmonary embolus is not an uncommon event but is difficult to diagnose in a bedridden ICU patient and especially difficult to diagnose on a portable ICU chest film.[127] There are many predisposing factors for a patient to develop a pulmonary embolus, including venous or cardiac disease, obesity, malignancy, dehydration, and the pill. Pulmonary emboli are also frequent in patients who have had hip, oncologic and prostate surgery. Occasionally, when classical clinical features are present, one can suggest the diagnosis.

The chest radiograph may be normal or most often demonstrates nonspecific changes, such as patchy infiltrates or changes in volume. The infiltrates tend to be peripheral, and one should remember that a pulmonary embolus does not usually present with recognizable radiographic appearances, except in the infrequent number of infants in whom an area of oligemia is present. Occasionally, one can discern a fairly classic abnormality such as classic Hampton hump,[128] which is a pleural-based triangular density with the apex oriented toward the hilum (Fig. 9.1).

ICU Chest Radiology: Principles and Case Studies, by Harold Moskowitz
Copyright © 2010 John Wiley & Sons, Inc.

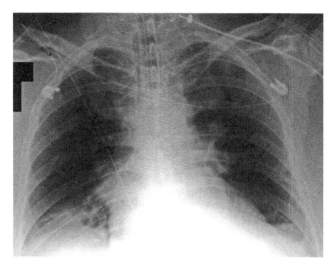

Figure 9.1   The triangular density abutting the right diaphragmatic pleura is the classic appearance of a Hampton hump.

This is due to an area of pulmonary infarction secondary to the embolis. Remember, many cases of pulmonary emboli do not produce associated infarction. Effusions occur in about 50% of patients who have pulmonary infarcts, and they are generally associated with the patient's developing chest pain. When an infarct has developed, this area does not tend to change rapidly, and one occasionally can distinguish among other causes of peripheral infiltrates due to edema or hemorrhage that do change fairly rapidly.

Fat embolism occurs when a large bone fractures and is also occasionally seen with pancreatitis, severe burns, or acute fatty liver. Neutral triglycerides are transported into the lungs where lipase hydrolyses into chemically active fatty acids that cause congestion, edema, intravascular coagulation, and, ultimately, alveolar hemorrhage. Chest x-rays are often normal in patients with small fat emboli, but with more extensive emboli a peripheral opacity can be seen. This occurs typically 1–3 days after trauma. There are other etiologies that cause pulmonary emboli, such as septic emboli from either an infected tricuspid valve or from intravenous drug injection. Also, occasionally, one can see amniotic fluid emboli from the uterus. Septic emboli most commonly are secondary to IV drug abusers or,

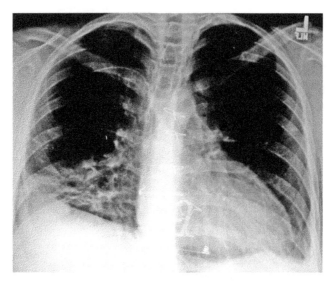

Figure 9.2   After tricuspid valve replacement surgery for endocarditis, the patient developed a clot on the valve and an embolus to the right lower lobe. Smaller emboli are presented on the left.

occasionally, in immunodepressed patients. Patients with infected endocarditis on the tricuspid valve often develop small, multiple emboli throughout both lung fields. *Staphylococcus aureus* and streptococci are the organisms most commonly involved.

The chest x-ray reveals nodular opacities, which are of multiple sizes, often have somewhat irregular borders, and often reveal cavity formation in these nodules.

Until recently, the radioisotope perfusion scan was the most sensitive, although nonspecific, diagnostic test for establishing pulmonary embolus (Fig. 9.2).[129] Abnormal perfusion, in an area of normal ventilation was the hallmark of the diagnosis of a positive scan. In the ICU patient, most had areas of this so-called mismatch, making the scan an unreliable test and necessitating the use of pulmonary angiography as a way to positively establish a diagnosis.[130]

With the advent of helical and multislice CT technology, the computerized tomography angiogram (CTA)[131] has replaced the radionuclide scan as a preferential way of establishing diagnosis.[132] Often it is very difficult to make the diagnosis, but the finding of a

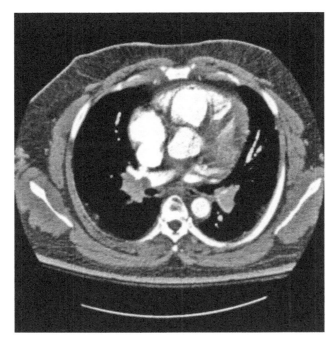

Figure 9.3 CTA reveals large pulmonary emboli bilaterally.

filling defect in the pulmonary vessel establishes it without question (Fig. 9.3).

PULMONARY HEMORRHAGE

Pulmonary hemorrhage and massive hemoptysis are very serious complications in an ICU patient.[133] If not correctly identified and treated they are often the cause of the patient's death. There are many causes of pulmonary hemorrhage, and imaging serves as the diagnostic test to identify the potential site of the bleed. Common causes of pulmonary hemorrhage include bronchiectosis, trauma, and inflammatory aneurysms (such as are seen in tuberculosis cavities). Other entities, such as bronchial tumors, idiopathic pulmonary hemorrhage, and Goodpasture syndrome should also be considered. If the underlying lung is normal, pulmonary hemorrhage will clear fairly rapidly within several days.

CHAPTER 10

ATELECTASIS AND COLLAPSE

Atelectasis is a very common cause of pulmonary disorders in the ICU.[134] It is often seen in patients after thoracic or upper abdominal surgery.[135] It is much more common in patients who have underlying lung problems and/or in smokers, elderly patients, and obese individuals.[136]

There are several mechanisms that cause atelectasis in adults, including obstructive, passive, compressive, and cicatricial etiologies. Another form of atelectasis, so-called adhesive atelectasis, is common in premature neonatal infants, secondary to insufficient production of surfactin.

The most common cause of atelectasis is obstruction. Acute endobronchial obstruction from mucus plugs is ubiquitous in the ICU population.[137] Decreased cough reflex and an inability to clear secretions, as well as sedation, intubation, and the usual supine position of these patients are all contributing factors. Impaired mucociliary function, increased secretions, and altered consciousness also contribute. Mucus plugging is the most common cause of acute segmental, lobar, or complete lung collapse (Fig. 10.1). Air bronchograms

ICU Chest Radiology: Principles and Case Studies, by Harold Moskowitz
Copyright © 2010 John Wiley & Sons, Inc.

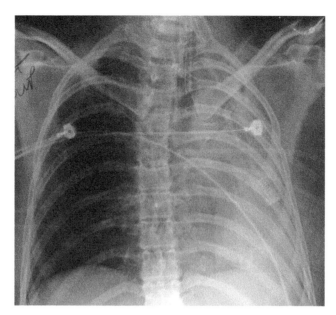

Figure 10.1   The complete collapse of the left lung with shift of the mediastinum to the left and elevation of the left hemidiaphragm due to endobronchial obstruction secondary to a large mucus plug.

are absent when the obstruction is in the proximal part of a large central airway. The absence of an air bronchogram, in patients who have acute lobar collapse, favors mucoid impaction as the cause, and often broncoscopy is the best method to treat these patients.[138]

Even in patients who are on mechanical ventilation, obstructive atelectasis can occur very rapidly. One theory is that highly oxygenated air, as opposed to normal ambient air, is quickly absorbed into the alveolar capillaries from the alveoli, so that collapse occurs within minutes.

Passive atelectasis is very often encountered in the ICU patient due to pleural effusions. Pneumothorax is also a cause of passive atelectasis. The lung tends to collapse on itself especially in the most dependent regions, where the effects of gravity help the effusion compress the lung. Thus partial lobar consolidations are more often seen in the lower lobe, particularly on the left, and are seen only occasionally in the upper lobes. The radiographic hallmark of this collapse is disappearance of the diaphragm, and it is important to

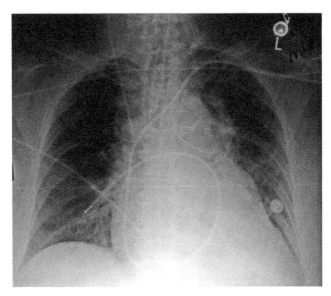

Figure 10.2 A portable film reveals an enlarged heart with left atrial enlargement. Note the atelectasis and collapse of the left lower lobe. The Swan-Ganz catheter is too far out into the right lower lobe bronchus.

differentiate atelectasis from effusion. Look for the presence of an air bronchogram, which is typical of this type of atelectasis. A CT will also demonstrate a homogeneous consolidation with a central air bronchogram.

Compressive atelectasis may be seen secondary to a preexisting mass, either a tumor or an abscess. These causes are somewhat unusual and the most common cause of compressive atelectasis is pleural fluid.

Many areas in the lung are can become atelectatic, but the left lower lobe is by far the most common site. Atelectasis of the right lower lobe occurs about a third less often than in the left lower lobe, and collapse of the right upper lobe occurs approximately 50% less than in the right lower lobe.

Collapse of the left lower lobe may be due to phrenic nerve injury, but most often occurs due to an enlarged left atrium, which compresses the left lower lobe bronchus (Fig. 10.2).[139]

Cicatricial atelectasis is volume loss secondary to pulmonary fibrosis and is most commonly seen in patients with underlying

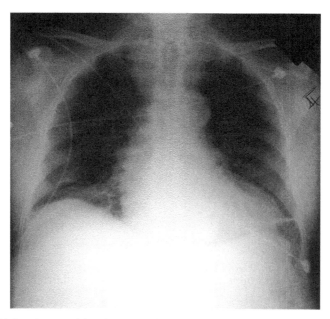

Figure 10.3   A portable film reveals a classic area of plate-like atelectasis in the region of the left lower lobe.

pulmonary disease. Often, this is seen in patients who develop significant pulmonary fibrosis as a late complication of ARDS.

The radiographic appearance of atelectasis depends on the extent and the location of the volume loss. Peripheral subsegmental atelectasis presents as linear densities predominately in the lung bases. This produces the so-called linear or plate-like atelectasis (Fig. 10.3).

Triangular or wedge-shaped opacities are secondary to a collapse of a bronchopulmonary segment. On a portable chest x-ray it may be difficult to differentiate lobar atelectasis from a segmental area of atelectasis with associated pneumonia, especially if signs of volume loss are not apparent (Fig. 10.4). Both can appear as areas of consolidation with air bronchograms, as long as there is no obstructive cause. The clinician will need to rely on clinical signs to distinguish between the two. Even then, differentiation is difficult because it does not take long for an area of atelectasis to become infected, resulting in fever and an elevated white count.

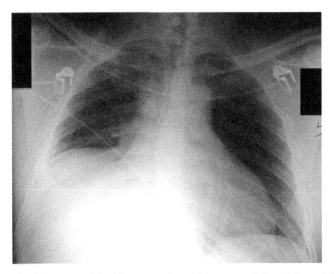

Figure 10.4   The portable film reveals atelectasis of the right middle and lower lobes.

CT is often helpful because it is easier to see volume loss on the CT scan than on the chest radiograph. It may be helpful to remember that in segmental atelectasis producing consolidation, the bronchi tend to be crowded together. Consolidation produced by pneumonia occupies space, does not crowd the bronchi, and does not often affect the volume of the lobe.

Occasionally an entire lobe may collapse. This will result in displacement of the intralobar fissure toward the area of collapse and a decrease in the lung volume of the affected lung. There will also be crowding of the bronchovascular markings. Compensatory expansion of adjacent lobes occurs, and there may be displacement and a shift of structures, such as the diaphragm, mediastinum, heart, or trachea.

Collapse of a lobe of the lung often has a characteristic appearance. In right upper lobe collapse, the minor fissure shifts superiorly, and the entire lobe shifts medially, presenting with a convex shadow abutting the superior vena cava.[140]

Right middle lobe collapse may sometimes be difficult to appreciate on the AP film, although one should look for the obliteration of

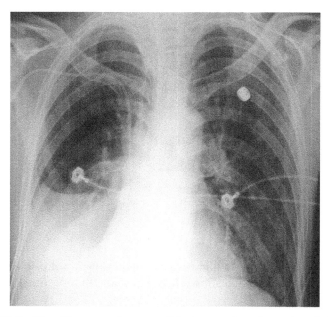

Figure 10.5   The film reveals consolidation and atelectasis of the right lower lobe. Note the obliteration of the right hemidiaphragm but persistence of the right heart border, indicating the right middle lobe is aerating normally.

the right cardiac shadow (Fig. 10.5). Normally, the right cardiac border is seen due to air in the right middle lobe.

The difference in density between the air in the right middle lobe acini and the tissue density of the heart results in an identifiable cardiac border. Loss of aeration of the middle lobe due either to complete collapse or filling of the acini with fluid, results in there being no difference in radiologic density between these two structures. Thus the cardiac shadow is no longer identifiable, the so-called silhouette sign.

A lateral film will often disclose the downward displacement of the minor fissure and the anterior displacement of the major fissure, with consolidation of the middle lobe (Fig. 10.6).[141]

The left upper lobe collapses in a characteristic appearance, with the major fissure shifting anteriorly, a phenomenon best seen on the lateral film. The AP film shows an upper mediastinum that increases in width medially, and there is obliteration of the left heart border.[142]

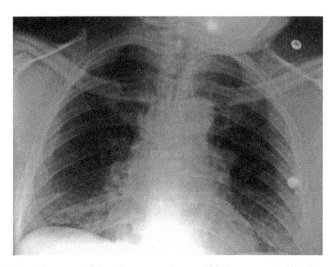

Figure 10.6   The portable film reveals a mild downward displacement of the horizontal fissure, indicating a loss of volume in a portion of the right lower lobe.

The lower lobes collapse posteriorly, causing the diaphragmatic shadow to be lost. In complete collapse of the lower lobe, the major fissure moves posteriorly, and the lobe becomes a triangular density in the costophrenic angle.

Differentiation between collapse, air space consolidation, and pleural effusion is often essential when one has to manage the ICU patient. The identification of volume loss presenting as a shift of either the mediastinum or a fissure, crowding of bronchi, or the loss of the border of either the heart or the diaphragm may help establish the correct diagnosis or initiate either bronchoscopic suction or appropriate respiratory therapy.

BIBLIOGRAPHY

1. Marik PE, Janower NL. The impact of routine chest radiography on ICU management decisions: An observational study. Am J Crit Care 1997;6:95–98.
2. Strain DS, Kinasewitz GT, Vereen LE. Value of routine of daily chest x-rays in the medical intensive care unit. Crit Care Med 1985; 13:534–536.
3. MacMahon H, Vyborny C. Technical advances in chest radiography. Am J Radiol 1994;163:1049–1059.
4. Tocino I. Chest imaging in the intensive care unit. Eur J Radiol 1996;23:46–57.
5. Barnes GT. Contrast in scatter and x-ray imaging. RadioGraphics 1991;11:307–323.
6. Floyd C, Baker JA, Lo JY, et al. Measurements of scatter fraction in clinical bedside radiography. Radiology 1992;183:857–861.
7. O'Donovan PB, Skipper GJ, Litchney JC, et al. Device for facilitating precise alignment in bedside radiography. Radiology 1992;184: 284–285.

8. Comeau WJ, White PD. A critical analysis of standard methods of estimating heart size from roentgen measurements. Am J Roentgen Radiol Ther 1942;47:665–667.

9. Fischer MR, Mintzer RA, Rogers LF, et al. Evaluation of a new mobile automatic exposure control device. Am J Radiol 1982; 139:1055–1059.

10. Korhola O, Bondestams S, Savikurki S, et al. Improvement of bedside chest radiography quality using a high radio grid and an electronic angle meter for alignment. Acta Radiol 1994;35:244–246.

11. Lo JY, Floyd CE, Ravin CE. Scatter compensation in chest radiography with a single exposure estimation subtraction method. Radiology 1990;177:172.

12. O'Donovan PB, Skipper GJ, Litchney JC, et al. Device for facilitating precise alignment in bedside radiography. Radiology 1992;184: 284–285.

13. Pandit-Bhalla M, Diethelm L, Espenan G. Portable chest radiographs in the intensive care units: Referral patterns and estimated cumulative radiation exposure. J Thorac Imaging 2002;17:211–213.

14. Chotas H, Floyd JCE, Ravin C. Technical evaluation of the digital chest radiography system that uses a selenium detector. Radiology 1995;195:264–270.

15. Schaefer C, Prokop M. Storage phosphor radiography of the chest. Radiology 1993;186:314–315.

16. Radfern R, Kundel HL, Polanksy M, et al. A picture archival and communication system shortens delays in obtaining radiographic information in the medical intensive care unit. Crit Care Med 2000;28:1231–1232.

17. Humfrey LM, Fitzpatrick K, Paine SS, Raven CE. Physician experience with viewing digital radiographs in an ICU environment. J Digit Imaging 1993;6:30–36.

18. Kundel HL, Seshadri SP, Langlotz CT, et al. Prospective study of a PACS: Information flow and clinical action in a medical intensive care unit. Radiology 1996;199:143–149.

19. Krivopal N, Shlobin OA, Schwartzstein RN. Utility of daily routine portable chest radiographs in mechanically ventilated patients in the medical ICU. Chest 2003;123:1607–1614.

20. Goodman LR, Conrady TA, Liang F. Radiographic evaluation of endotracheal tube position. Am J Radiol 1976;127:433–434.

21. Lotan OR, Gerber D, Aserom S, Santarelli R. Utility of post intubation chest radiographs in the ICU. Crit Care 2000;4:50–53.

22. Conrardy TA, Goodman LR, Lainge R, Singer NN. Alteration of endotracheal tube position—Flexion and extension of the neck. Crit Care Med 1976;4:7–14.

23. Stauffer JL, Olsen DE, Petty TL. Complications and consequences of endotracheal intubation and tracheotomy: A prospective study of 150 critically ill adult patients. Am J Med 1991;70:65–68.

24. Khan F, Reddy N, Khan A. Cuff-trachea ratio as an indicator of tracheal damage. Chest 1976;70:431–432.

25. Smith GN, Reed JC, Chaplin RH. Radiographic detection of esophageal malpositioning of endotracheal tube. Am J Radiol 1990; 154:23–24.

26. Khan F, Reddy NC. Enlarging intratracheal tube cuff diameter; A quantitative rentgenographic study of its value in the early prediction of serious tracheal damage. Ann Thorac Surg 1977, 24:49–53.

27. Greenbaum DM, Marshall LKE. The value of routine daily chest x-rays in intubated patients in the medical intensive care units. Crit Care Med 1982;10:29.

28. Wechler RJ, Steiner RM, Kinori T. Monitoring the monitors: the radiology of thoracic catheters, wires and tubes. Semin Roentgenol 1988;23:61–84.

29. Rollins RJ, Tocino I. Early radiographic signs of tracheal rupture. Am J Rentgenol 1987;148:695–698.

30. Gray P, Sullivan G, Ostryznick P, et al. Value of post procedural chest radiographs in adult intensive care unit. Crit Care Med 1992; 20:1513–1518.

31. Sivak SL, Hummel. Late appearance of pneumothrax after subclavian venapuncture. Am J Med 1986;80:323–324.

32. Yilnazlar A, Bilgin H, Korfali G. Complications of 1303 central venous cannulations. J R Soc Med 1998;90:319–321.

33. Conces DJ, Holden RW. Aberrant locations and complications in initial placement of subclavian vein catheters. Arch Surg 1984; 119:293–295.

34. Tocino IM, Watanabe A. Impending catheter perforation of super vena cava: Radiographic recognition. Am J Radiol 1986;146: 487–492.

35. Hunt R, Hunter TD. Cardiac tamponade and deaths from perforation of the right atrium via central venous catheter. Am J Radiol 1988; 151:1250–1252.

36. Demos T, Posniak IT, Pierce K, et al. Venous aomalies of the thorax. Am J Radiol 2000;182:1139–1150.

37. Clarke DE, Raffin TA. Infectious complications of long term indwelling central venous catheters. Chest 1990;97:966–972.
38. Fischer J, Lundstrom J, Ottander H. Central venous cannulation—A radiologic determination of catheter positions and immediate intrathoracic complications. Acta Anaesthesiol Scand 1977;21:45049.
39. Miller KS, Sahn SA. Chest tubes: Indications, technique, management and complications. Chest 1987;91:258–264.
40. Webb WR, LaBerge JN. Radiographic recognition of chest tube malposition in the major fissure. Chest 1984;85:81–88.
41. McConaghy PM, Kennedy N. Tension pneumothorax due to intrapulmonary placement of chest tube. Anaesth Intensive Care 1995; 23:496–498.
42. Miller WT, Tino G, Fredburg JS. Thoracic CT in the intensive care unit: Assessment of clinical usefulness. Radiology 1998;209:491–498.
43. Ghahremani GG, Gould RJ. Nasoenteric feeding tubes: Radiographic detection of complications. Dig Dis Sci 1986;31:574–585.
44. Owen RL, Cheney FW. Endobronchial intubation: A preventable complication. Anesthesiology 1987;67:255–257.
45. Woodall BH, Winfield DF, Bisset GS. Inadvertent tracheobronchial placement of feeding tubes. Radiology 1975;116:19–25.
46. McLoud TC, Putman C. Radiology of Swan Ganz catheter and associated pulmonary complications. Radiology 1975;116:19–25.
47. Sise MJ, Hollingsworth P, Brinn JE. Complications of the flow directed pulmonary artery catheter. A perspective analysis of 219 patients. Crit Care Med 1981;9:315.
48. Chang CF. Esophageal rupture due to Sengstaken-Blakemore tube placement. World J gastroenterol 2005;11(41):6563–6565 (Nov).
49. Vlavianos P, Gimson AE, Westaby D, et al. Balloon tamponade in variceal bleeding: use and misuse. BMJ 1989;298:1158.
50. Hyson EA, Ravin CE, Kelley MJ. The intra-aortic counter pulsation balloon: radiographic considerations. Am J Radiol 1977;128:915–919.
51. Karlson KD, Martin EC, Bregman D. Superior mesenteric artery obstruction by intra-aortic counter pulsation balloon simulating embolism. Cardiovasc Intervent Radiol 1981;4:236–238.
52. Beckman CB, Geha AS, Hammond GL. Results and complications of intraaortic balloon counterpulsation. Ann Thoracic Surg 1977; 24:550–559.
53. Daly BD, Cascade PN, Hummel JD. Transvenous and subcutaneous implantable cardioverter defibrillators: Radiographic assessment. Radiology 1994;191:273–278.

54. DeBeBiulir M, Kanver C. Twiddler's syndrome. Complicating a trans-venous defibrillator lead. Chest 1996;109:1391–1394.

55. Tocino I, Wescott JL. Barotrauma. Radiol Clin North Am 1996; 34:59–81.

56. Gammon RB, Shin MS, Groves RH, et al. Clinical risk factors for pulmonary barotrauma: A multivariate analysis. Am J Respir Crit Care Med 1995;152(4):1235–1240.

57. Marini JJ, Colver BH, Butler J. Mechanical effect of lung distention with positive pressure on cardiac function. Ann Rev Respir Dis 1981;124:382–386.

58. Raptopoulous Z, Davis LM, Lee G. Factors effecting the development of pneumothrax associated with thoracentesis. Am J Radiol 1991; 156:917–920.

59. Ziter FM, Westcott JL. Supine sub-pulmonary pneumothrax. Am J Radiol 1981;137:699–701.

60. Tocino IM. Pneumothrax in the supine patient: Radiographic anatomy. Radiographics 1985;5:557–586.

61. Gordon R. A Deep sulcus sun. Radiology 1980;30:25–27.

62. Tocino IM, Miller MH, Fairfax WR. Distribution of pneumothrax in a supine and semirecumbent critically ill adult. Am J Radiol 1985; 144:901–905.

63. Kollef NH. Risk factors for the misdiagnosis of pneumothrax in the intensive care unit. Crit Care Med 1991;19:906–910.

64. Tsuno K, Prato T, Kolobow T. Acute lung injury from mechanical ventilation and moderately high airway pressures. J Appl Physiol 1990;69:956–961.

65. Zwilich CW, Pierson DJ, Creagh CE, et al. Complications of assisted ventilation: A prospective study of 354 consecutive episodes. Am J Med 1974;57:161–169.

66. Steier N, Ching N, Roberts E, Nealno T. Pneumothrax complicating continuous rentaltory support. J Thorac Cardiovasc Surg 1974; 67:17–23.

67. Fewell JE, Abendshcein DR, Carlson CJ. Mechanism of decreased right and left ventricular endystolic volumes during continuous posi-tive ventilation. Circ Res 1980;47:467–471.

68. Dreyfuss D, Soler P, Bassett G. High inflation pressure pulmonary edema. Respective effects of high airway pressure, high tidal volume, and positive end expiratory pressure. Am Rev Respir Dis 1988; 137:1159–1164.

69. Pierson DJ. Alveolar rupture during mechanical ventilation: Role of PEEP peak airway pressure and distending volume. Respir Care 1988;33:472–478.
70. McLaud TC, Baolash PG, Rabin CE. PEEP: Radiographic features and associated complications. Am J Radiol 1977;129:209–214.
71. Leeming BWA. Radiologic aspects of pulmonary complications resulting from intermittent positive pressure ventilation. Austral Radiol 1978;12:361–363.
72. Zylak CM, Standen JR, Barnes GR. Pneumomediastinum revisited. Radiographics 2000;20:1043–1057.
73. Cyrlak D, Milne ENC, Imray TJ. Pneumomediastinum: A diagnostic problem. Crit Rev Diagn Imaging 1984;23:75–79.
74. Lebin B. The continuous diaphragm sign. A newly recognized sign of pneumomediastinum. Clin Radiol 1973;24;337–339.
75. Gilbert TB, McGrath BJ. Tension Pneumothrax: Etiology, diagnosis, pathophysiology and management. J Intensive Care Med 1994; 9:139–144.
76. Grosfeld JL, Kilman JW. Frye TR. Spontaneous pneumopericardium in the newborn infant. J Pediat 1970;76:614–616.
77. Johnson TH, Atman AR. Pulmonary interstitial gas: First sign of barotrauma due to PEEP therapy. Crit Care Med 1979;7:532–536.
78. Boothroyd AE, Barson AJ. Pulmonary interstitial emphysema: A radiologic pathologic correlation. Pediatr Radiol 1988;18:194–197.
79. Tocino I, Wescott JL. Barotrauma. Rad Clin North Am 1996;34: 59–81.
80. Ruiz-Santana S, Garcia JA, Esteban. ICU pneumonias: A multi-institutional study. Crit Care Med 1987;15:930–935.
81. Lipchik RJ, Kuzo RS. Nosocomial pneumonia. Radiol Clin North Am 1996;94:47–57.
82. George DL. Epidemiology of nosocomial pneumonia in intensive care unit patients. Clin Chest Med 1995;16:29–44.
83. Drikx MR, Craven DE, Celli BR, et al. Nosocomial pneumonia in intubated patients given sucralfate as compared with antacids or histamine Type II blockers. The role of gastric colonization. JEGM. 1987;317:1376–1382.
84. Goularte TA, Lictenberg DA, Craden DE. Gastric colonization in patients receiving antacids and mechanical ventilation: A mechanism for pharyngeal colonization. Am J Infect Control 1986;14:88–91.
85. VonBaum H, Ewig S, Marre R, et al. Competence network for community acquired pneumonia (*Legionella* pneumonia) study group. Clin Infect Dis 2008;46:1355–1364.

86. Chan CK, Hyland RH, Hutcheon MA. Pulmonary complications following bone marrow transplantation. Clin Chest Med 1990;11: 323–339.
87. Azouolay E, Timset J, Taffler, et al. *Candida* colonization of the respiratory tract and subsequent *Pseudomonas* ventilator-associated pneumonia. Chest 2006;129:110–117.
88. Cook DJ, Walter SD, Cook RJ, et al. Incidents of and risk factors for ventilator associated pneumonia in critically ill patients. Ann Intern Med 1999;130:1027–1028.
89. Wunderink RG, Oldenberg LS, Zeiss J. The radiologic diagnosis of autopsy proven ventilator associated pneumonia. Chest 1992;101: 458–463.
90. Estes RJ, Meduri GU. The pathogenesis of ventilator associated pneumonia: Mechanisms of bacterial transcolinization and airway inoculation. Intensive Care Med 1985;21:356–383.
91. Torres A, Al EL, Ebialy M, Padro L. Validation of different techniques for the diagnosis of ventilator associated pneumonia. Am J Respir Crit Care Med 1994;149:324–331.
92. Maduri GU, Mauldin GL, Wunderink RG, et al. Causes of dyspnea and pulmonary densities in patients with clinical manifestations of ventilator associated pneumonia. Chest 1994;106:221–235.
93. Winer-Muram HT, Ruben SA, Ellis JV. Pneumonia and ARDS in patients receiving mechanical ventilation: Diagnostic accuracy of chest radiography. Radiology 1993;188:479–485.
94. Kollef NH, Schuster DP. Ventilator associated pneumonia: clinical considerations. Am J Radiol 1994;163:1031–1035.
95. Hershey CO, Panaro D. Round pneumonia in adults. Arch Inern Med 1988;148:1155–1157.
96. Hamer DH. Treatment of nosocomial pneumonia and trachea bronchitis caused by multi-drug resistant pseudomonias with aerosoliged colistin. Am J Respir Crit Care Med 2000;162:328–330.
97. McLoud TC, Naidich DP. Thoracic disease in immunocompromised patient. Radiol Clin North Am 1992;30:525–542.
98. Buff SJ, McClelland R, Gallis HA. *Candida albicans* pneumonia. Am J Radiol 1982;138:645–650.
99. Han D, SooLee K, Franquet T. Thrombotic and nonthrombotic pulmonary arterial embolism: spectrum of imaging findings. Radiographics 2003;23:1521–1593.
100. Chan CK, Hyland RH, Hutcheon MA. Pulmonary complications following bone marrow transplantation. Clin Chest Med 1990;11: 323–339.

101. Milne E. Hydrostatic versus increased permeability pulmonary edema. Radiology 1989;170:891–892.

102. Milne ENC, Pistolesi N. Reading the Chest Radiograph: A Physiologic Approach. Mosby Yearbook: Chapter 4; St. Louis 1993.

103. Staub MC. The pathogenesis of pulmonary edema. Prog Cardiovasc Dis 1980;23:53–58.

104. Sibbald WJ, Cunningham DR, Chin DN. Noncardiac or cardiac pulmonary edema? A practical approach to clinical differentiation in critically ill patients. Chest 1983;84:452–457.

105. Aberle DR, Winer-Kronish JP, Webb WR. Hydrostatic versus increased permeability pulmonary edema: Diagnosis based on radiographic criteria in critically ill patients. Radiology 1998;168:73–79.

106. Milne ENC, Pistolesi N, Minati N, Giuntini C. A radiologic distinction of cardiogenic and non-cardiogenic edema. Am J Radiol 1985;144: 879–894.

107. Duane PG, Colice GL. Impact of noninvasive studies to distinguish volume overload from ARDS in acutely ill patients with pulmonary edema: Analysis of the medical literature from 1966 to 1998. Chest 2000;118:1709–1717.

108. Woodring JH, Given CH. Noninvasive estimator of pulmonary wedge pressure. Am J Respir Crit Care Med 2000;161:85–90.

109. Chakko S, Woska D, Martinez H. Clinical, radiographic and hemodynamic correlations in chronic congestive failure. Am J Med 1991; 90:353–359.

110. Milne ENC, Pistoloesi N, Miniati N, Giuntini C. The vascular pedicle of the heart and vena amicus, part one: The normal subject. Radiology 1984;152:108.

111. Milne ENC, Pistoloesi N, Miniati N, Giuntini C. The vascular pedicle of the heart and vena azygous: Acquired heart disease. Radiology 1984;152:9–17.

112. Badgett R, Mulrow C, Otto P. How well can the chest radiograph diagnose left ventricular dysfucntion? J Gen Intern Med 1996; 11:625–634.

113. Elyi WE, Smith AC, Chiles C, et al. Radiologic determination of intravascular volume status using portable digital chest radiograph: A perspective investigation in 100 patients. Crit Care Med 2001; 29:1502–1512.

114. Wandtke J. Bedside chest radiography. Radiology 1994;190:1–10.

115. Conen A, Ladina J, Bigisser R. Ipsilateral re-expansion pulmonary edema after drainage of a spontaneous pneumothorax. J Med Case Reports 2007;1:107–110.

116. Lichtenstein D, Meziere G. A lung ultrasound sign allowing bedside distinction between pulmonary edema and COPD: The comet tail artifact. Intensive Care Med 1998;24:1331–1334.

117. Ketai LH, Godwin JD. State of the art: A new view of pulmonary edema and respiratory distress syndrome. J Thoracic Imaging 1998;13:147–171.

118. Ashbaugh DG, Bigelow DB, Petty TL. Acute respiratory distress in adults. Lancet 1967;2:319–323.

119. Matthay MA, Zimmerman GA. Acute lung injury and the acute respiratory distress syndrome: Four decades of inquiry into pathogenesis and rational management. Ann J Respir Cell Nal Biol 2005; 33:319–327.

120. Goodman LR. Congestive heart failure and adult respiratory distress syndrome. Rad Clin North Am 1996;34:33–46.

121. Greene R. Adult respiratory distress syndrome: Acute alveola damage. Radiology 1987;163:57–66.

122. Schuster DP. What is lung injury? What is ARDS? Chest 1995; 107:1721–1726.

123. Gattinoni L, D'Andrea L, Pelosi P, et al. Regional effects in mechanism of positive end expiratory pressure in early adult respiratory distress syndrome. J Am Med Assoc 1993;269:2122–2127.

124. Maunder RJ, Shuman WT, McHugh JW. Preservation of normal lung regions in the adult respiratory distress syndrome: Analysis by computer tomography. J Am Med Assoc 1986;255:2463–3469.

125. Gattinoni L, Caironi P, Cressoni M. Lung recruitment in patients with the acute respirtatory distress syndrome. N Engl J Med 2006; 354:1775–1786.

126. Montgomery AB, Stager MA, Carrico CJ, Hudson LD. Causes of mortality in patients with adult respiratory distress syndrome. Am Rev Respir 1985;132:485–489.

127. Anderson FA, Wheeler HB, Goldberg RJ. A population based perspective of hospital incidence and case fatality rates of venous thrombosis and pulmonary embolis. Arch Intern Med 1991;153:933–948.

128. Hampton AD. Hampton hump. Am J Radiol 1940;43:305–309.

129. PIEPED Investigators. Value of ventilation (perfusion) scan in acute pulmonary embolism: Results of prospective investigation of pulmonary embolism diagnosis. J Am Med Assoc 1990;263:2753–2759.

130. Remy-Jardin N, Remy J, Wattinne L, Giraud F. Central pulmonary thromboembolism: diagnosis via spiral volumetric ct with the single

breath hold technique: Comparison with pulmonary angiography. Radiology 1992;185:381–387.

131. Ghaye B, Ghuysen A, Bruyene PJ, et al. Can CT pulmonary angiography allow assessment of severity and prognosis in patients with pulmonary embolism? What the radiologist needs to know. Radiographics 2005;26:23–40.

132. Gefter W, Hatabu H, Highland G. State of the art pulmonary thromboembolism: Recent developments in diagnosis using compiled tomography and magnetic resonance imaging. Radiology 1995;197:562–574.

133. Crocco JA, Rooney JJ, Frankunshen DS. Massive hemoptysis. Arch Intern Med 1968;121:495–498.

134. Siegel MD, Tocino I. Chest radiology in the intensive care unit. Clin Pulmon Med 1999;6:347–355.

135. Sheuland JE, Hirleleman MR, Hoang AA. Lobar collapse in the surgical intensive care unit. Br J Radiol 1983;56:531–534.

136. Gale GD, Teasdale SJ, Sanders DE. Pulmonary atelectasis and other respirator complications after cardiopulmonary bypass and investigation of etiologic factors. Can Anaesth Soc J 1979;26:15–21.

137. Pham DH, Huang D, Korwan A. Acute unilateral pulmonary non ventilatoin due to mucous plugs. Radiology 1987;165:135–137.

138. Kreider NE, Lipson DA. Bronchoscopy for atelectasis in the ICU: Case report and review of the literature. Chest 2003;24:344–350.

139. Benjamin J, Cascade P, Ruben Fire M. Left lower lobe atelectasis and consolidation following cardiac surgery. Radiology 1982;142:11–14.

140. Proto AZ, Tocino I. Radiographic manifestations of lobar collapse. Semin Roentgenol 1980;15:117–134.

141. Lee KS, Logan PM, Primack SL, Muller NL. Combined lobar atelectasis of the right lung: Imaging findings. Am J Radiol 1994; 163:43–67.

142. Mardenstrom B, Novek J. The atelectatic complex of the left lung. Acta Radiol 1960;3:173–184.

SECTION II

CASE STUDIES

TUBES, LINES, AND CATHETERS

CASE 1

This 48-year-old patient presented with a tumor in the tail of the pancreas. He underwent a distal pancreatectomy, which was complicated by lacerating the spleen. Several hours later in the ICU, he had increasing shortness of breath and a decrease in his oxygen saturation.

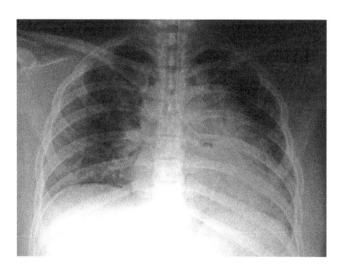

ICU Chest Radiology: Principles and Case Studies, by Harold Moskowitz
Copyright © 2010 John Wiley & Sons, Inc.

Discussion

As you looked at this film, you noticed, of course, the endotracheal tube malpositioned in the left mainstem bronchus. You also noticed the lack of definition of the left heart border and the increased density in the perihilar regions. You recognize that the endotracheal tube is occluding the lingular segment of the left upper lobe, indicating left upper lobe collapse, resulting in obliteration of the left heart border. The endotracheal tube was moved back into its proper position, approximately 4 cm above the carina, and the lingular segment of the left upper lobe reaerated.

CASE 2

This 68-year-old patient is now 3 days post cardiac bypass surgery and is doing very well. This film was taken after the patient had been extubated.

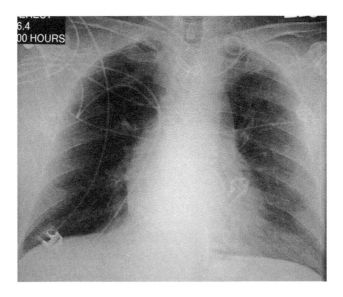

Discussion

The patient is doing extremely well and aerating well without an effusion. You do notice the coiling of the left subclavian central line.

Approximately 30% of all lines inserted are in poor position and need to be replaced.

CASE 3

This patient suddenly lost consciousness while visiting his wife in the hospital. He was brought to the emergency department, where it was discovered that he was in ventricular fibrillation, and he was resuscitated. He was then transferred to the cardiac catheterization laboratory.

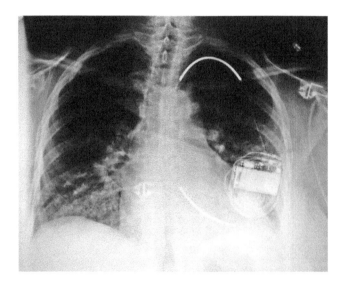

Discussion

This patient had what type of device inserted? You notice the somewhat peculiar position of the intraventricular cardiac defibrillator (ICD). First, it is worth remembering the characteristic appearance of this device. Note how it differs from a pacemaker. The distal end is thicker with a serrated area. Proximally, another wider serrated area, approximately 3 in. in length, is seen. These are the defibrillator parts of the ICD. In this patient, however, note the position of the device. What ventricle should this be in? It should be in the right ventricle, and here, in the haste and confusion surrounding this patient's care, it was unfortunately inserted in the arterial side, so that the ICD is in the apex of the left ventricle.

CASE 4

This 60-year-old female arrived in the hospital with a large right pleural effusion, which was tapped and discovered to be tuberculosis. A chest tube was placed to drain the effusion. The chest tube was not functioning well, and a portable film was obtained.

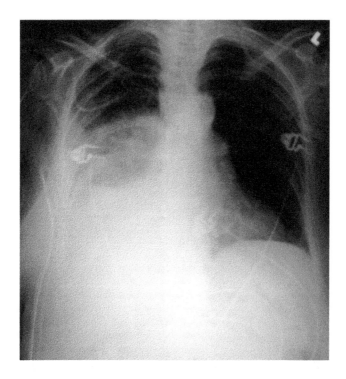

Discussion

In this film you can immediately identify the reason the chest tube is not functional. It is not in the pleural space but rather in the subcutaneous tissues. There is, on careful observation, some air in the subcutaneous tissue. Again note the large right effusion with compressive atelectasis. A central line is into the superior vena cava.

CASE 5

This 77-year-old patient presented to the emergency department in shock, with severe chest pain, having sustained a large anterolateral myocardial infarct. He was admitted to the ICU, where a Swan-Ganz catheter was placed. His wedge pressure was recorded during the night as 17 mm Hg, and you arrived in the morning to see this film.

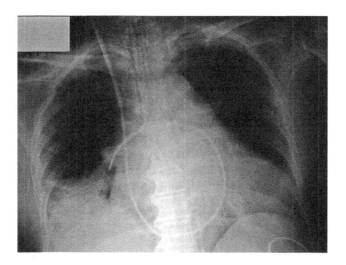

Discussion

The portable film reveals considerable cardiomegaly, and a Swan-Ganz catheter that was introduced via the right internal jugular route. Did you notice anything abnormal about the Swan-Ganz catheter? Of course, the catheter is placed too far peripherally into the right lower lobe pulmonary artery. Proper position should be in the right main pulmonary artery. In addition, if you look carefully at the tip, you can see that the balloon is still inflated. The balloon was inflated and was not deflated after the wedge pressure was obtained. A pulmonary infarct developed distal to the position of the catheter in the right lower lobe. There are two feared complications with the Swan-Ganz catheter, and this is one of them. In addition to thrombosis, there is always the danger that inflating the balloon at the tip of the Swan-Ganz catheter may cause a small pulmonary artery to rupture, and the patient will develop intrapulmonary hemorrhage.

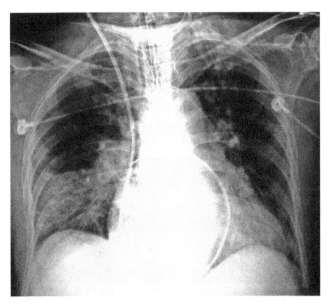

On this film, taken later, the catheter has been withdrawn into a normal position in the right main pulmonary artery, but the area of infarction is still seen.

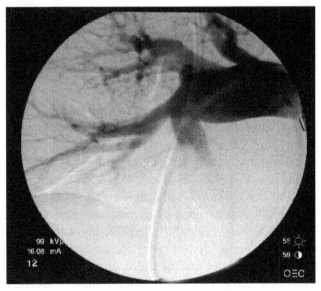

A film from the right selective pulmonary angiogram reveals the clot in the right lower pulmonary artery.

CASE 6

This 56-year-old patient is 1 day after what surgical procedure?

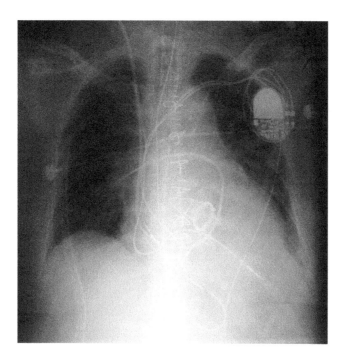

Discussion

The portable film is similar to many portable films taken in post-op patients. Of course, as you look, you can see that this patient has had bypass surgery with a left internal mammary artery bypass. You can identify this by seeing the clips all the way up to the left subclavian, indicating that the left internal mammary has been dissected. One can follow the clips down, probably to the region of the left anterior descending artery, where it was anastomosed. Of course, you recognize that this patient has had both a mitral and an aortic valve inserted. What tubes do you see? There is a Swan-Ganz catheter, which is well out into the main right pulmonary artery and probably should be pulled back approximately 2 cm. In addition, there is a right and a left chest tube, both in good position without a pneumothrax. There are two mediastinal drainage tubes, one in the upper mediastinum at approximately T6, and another lying inferiorly in the region of the pericardium.

There is one other rather significant finding on this film related to another tube. Do you see it?

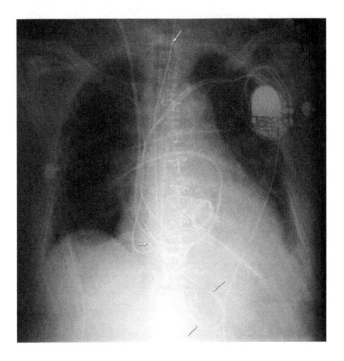

Of course you noticed the position of the NG tube proceeding down into the stomach, but coiling back into the distal end of the esophagus. This is unacceptable because aspiration can occur. There are two reasons to have a nasogastric tube in place. One is just for suction, and the tip and the side hole can be in the upper half of the stomach. If one is using the NG tube to feed a patient, it is preferable to have the tube either distal to the pylorus or close by. You also noticed that there is partial collapse of the left lower lobe. There is increased density and partial obscurity of the diaphragm, indicating collapse of a portion in the left lower lobe.

CASE 7

This 78-year-old man is 7 days post bypass surgery.

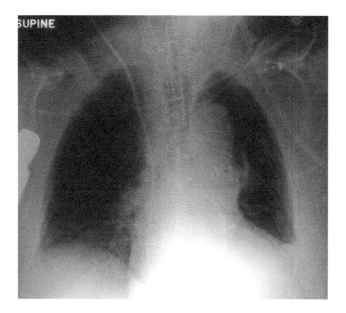

Discussion

As you look at this portable film, there are several things that should arouse your interest. First the Swan-Ganz, introduced via the internal jugular, is probably just out into the right main pulmonary artery and needs to be placed 3–4 cm farther out.

The endotracheal tube is interesting. Did you notice the air-containing area in the region of the thoracic outlet? This obviously is the cuff on the endotracheal tube, which has been blown up and is wider than the lumen of the trachea. The clinicians had problems keeping this patient, who has chronic obstructive lung disease, aerated. The balloon cuff was inflated and, initially, there was leaking around the cuff, so air was continuously added to the cuff, which is now overinflated. It is very important that this cuff be deflated every hour so as to prevent a major complication that can result postendotracheal intubation. The feared complication is stricture, secondary to fibrosis and scarring. This occurs either from erosions caused by the tube or, at times, from overdistention of the balloon, which produces a decrease in the vasculature to the mucosa of the trachea, with secondary ischemia, sloughing of the mucosa, fibrosis, scarring, and stricture.

Also note that the patient has a left effusion.

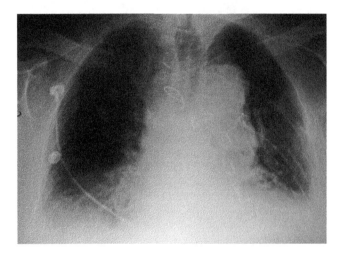

This film, taken approximately 4 days later, reveals that the endotracheal tube has been removed. The patient is still in failure and has a persistent left effusion. The Swan-Ganz has also been removed. Do you notice any other abnormality?

Note the changes in the position of the sternal wires. If you look back at the previous film, the wires were all lined up, one above another. Now there is peculiar placement of the wires, indicating that this patient has an infected sternum, and one should worry about the possibility of a sternal dehiscence.

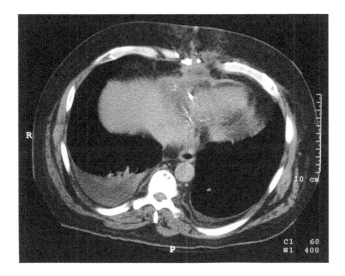

A CT scan was obtained, which revealed a collection in the region of the sternum, extending posteriorly. The patient was febrile, and aspiration revealed methycline-resistance *Staphylococcus aureus*.

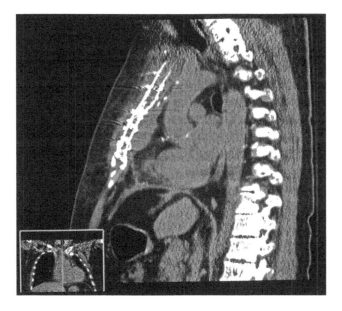

Sagital reconstruction reveals to better advantage the collection substernally. The patient was taken to the operating room.

CASE 8

This portable is of a 21-year-old patient immediately postoperative. Evaluate the film and see if you can determine what would lead the physicians to perform surgery on this patient.

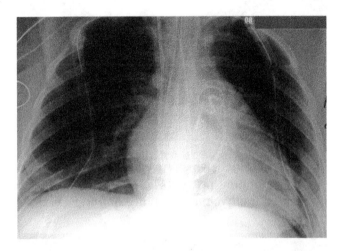

Discussion

The portable film reveals two chest tubes in good position. The patient obviously has had cardiac surgery. You did note, of course, that there were two artificial valves. They are somewhat unusual, in that one is in the aortic position and the other has a Swan-Ganz catheter going through it. This is an artificial pulmonic valve. It is quite unusual to have prosthetic valves inserted in a patient this young. However, the patient had extensive endocarditis with involvement of both the aortic and pulmonic valves, necessitating both of them to be replaced. In addition, there is a density, probably atelectasis, of the left lower lobe, posteriorly.

CASE 9

This patient has chronic obstructive lung disease and was admitted to the ICU in respiratory failure. The nurses noted his Po_2 was markedly decreased, and a portable chest x-ray was obtained.

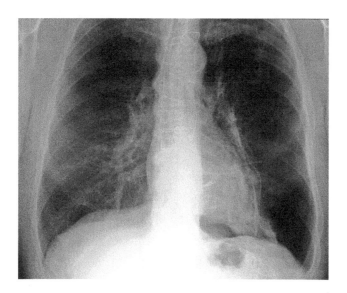

Discussion

This portable film reveals changes compatible with this patient's known COPD, with bullous changes in the apex. Note the changes in his sternum, secondary to infection, necessitating reconstruction of a portion of the sternum. At this time, however, the significant finding is the pneumothrax seen on the left, indicated by the lucency in the left costophrenic sulcus. This is an example of the so-called deep sulcus sign.

CASE 10

This 88-year-old man was in the hospital with multisystem failure, when he went into shock. An NG tube was placed and a film obtained.

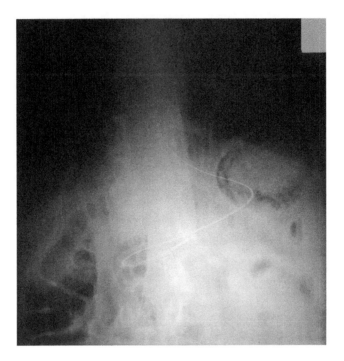

Discussion

A film centered at the diaphragm reveals the NG tube coiled back on itself. Did you notice the peculiar configuration to the gastric fundus? This represents air in the wall of the stomach, indicating necrosis of the wall of the stomach. This is similar to what happens with necrotizing entrocolitis.

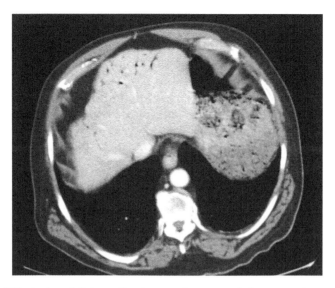

The CT study of this patient reveals to much better advantage the air in the wall of the stomach, as well as air in the portal venous system. This is a very poor prognostic sign.

CASE 11

This 56-year-old patient returned to the hospital with fever and chest pain. His previous history is significant: He had a carcinoma of the lung, necessitating a pneumonectomy 2 years earlier.

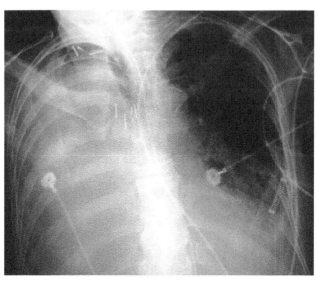

Discussion

This portable film reveals total opacification of the right hemithorax, secondary to this patient's pneumonectomy. Note the large metallic clips in the region of the right hilum.

You noticed, of course, the lack of definition in the left hemidiaphragm, and there is infiltrate and an air bronchogram in the left lower lobe, secondary to a pneumonia. What is particularly troublesome, however, is the fact that there is air in the apex of the right hemithorax. Can you think why this occurs? Unfortunately, there has been recurrent tumor at the stump of the right mainstem bronchus, with breakdown and air entering the pleural space. In addition, there is overflow infection into the left lower lobe, causing pneumonia.

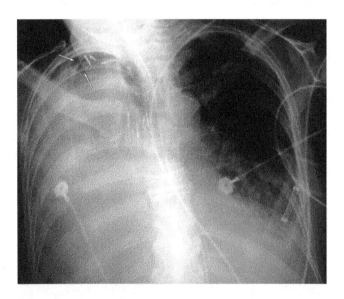

CASE 12

This 38-year-old patient was admitted to the ICU after he went into rapid atrial fibrillation. The portable was obtained before cardioverting this patient.

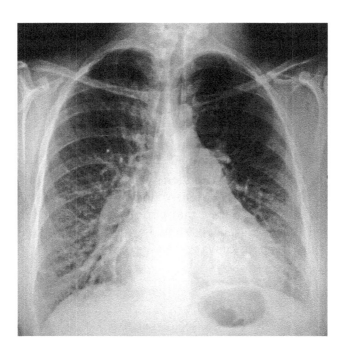

Discussion

The portable film reveals the heart to be somewhat enlarged. Of interest is the pulmonary vascularity. There is an enlarged pulmonary artery segment, as well as large pulmonary arteries and pulmonary veins. The waist of the heart is narrow, and findings are all consistent with the patient having a left to right shunt. While no lateral film was obtained, one can see that the left mainstem bronchus is not elevated, suggesting that the left atrium is normal. The three most common left to right shunts are atrial septal defect (ASD), ventricular septal defect (VSD), and patent ductus arteriosis. In a VSD, the left atrium is generally enlarged, whereas in a ASD, the atrium is small. The patient had an ASD, which was repaired.

BAROTRAUMA

CASE 13

This film is of a 68-year-old patient who had been in the ICU for approximately 2 weeks for extensive lower lobe aspiration pneumonia. He was intubated during that period of time, which eventually necessitated having a tracheostomy. This is the film taken immediately after the tracheostomy.

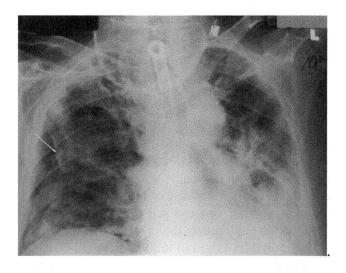

ICU Chest Radiology: Principles and Case Studies, by Harold Moskowitz
Copyright © 2010 John Wiley & Sons, Inc.

Discussion

The film now reveals persistent left lower lobe and left upper lobe pneumonia. Note the obliteration of most of the left cardiac border, secondary to the involvement of the inferior division of the lingular segment of the upper lobe. Of interest however, is the pneumothorax, which has developed on the right. This patient has long-standing interstitial fibrosis with a pneumonia now superimposed. As a result of a prolonged period on the respirator, he developed a pneumothorax, which is a common complication.

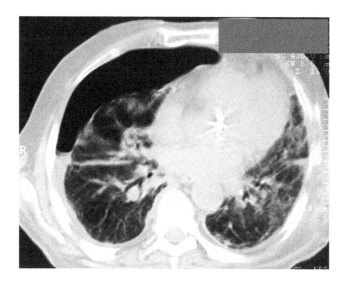

A CT study performed on this patient the following day reveals the extensive right-sided pneumothorax with a small right-sided effusion. The changes in the left lung are seen to better advantage on CT. CT is very sensitive for the evaluation of pneumothorax.

CASE 14

This 42-year-old female was admitted to the ICU, with marked dyspnea and shortness of breath, 2 days after spending a weekend on a farm, working in the barn. Her initial x-rays revealed alveolar densities at the periphery of both lungs, and the diagnosis of a euce-nephalic pneumonia was entertained. Her status necessitated that she be intubated. The film was taken 3 days later.

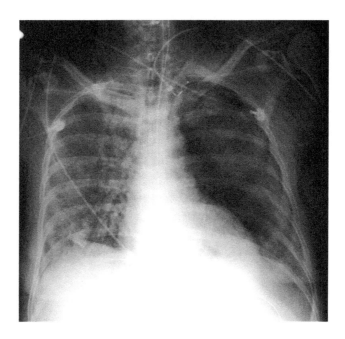

Discussion

This film reveals the infiltrate in both lung fields in the periphery consistent with an allergic pneumonitis. Note the pneumothorax on the left, secondary to dissection of air out of the alveoli, resulting in a pneumothorax.

CASE 15

This 82-year-old patient was admitted to the ICU due to marked shortness of breath caused by a marked decrease in Po_2. He was intubated, and a postintubation film was obtained.

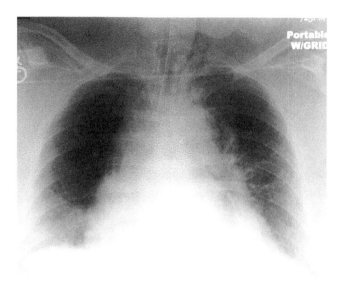

Discussion

You noticed, of course, the position of the endotracheal tube, which is just above the carina. There is considerable air in the mediastinum, extending up to the neck, representing mediastinal emphysema. Did you notice any other findings? The left hemidiaphragm is elevated, and there is an area of atelectasis in the left lower lobe.

CASE 16

This 82-year-old patient was admitted from the emergency department to the ICU, after extreme sharp chest pain and a marked decrease in oxygenation.

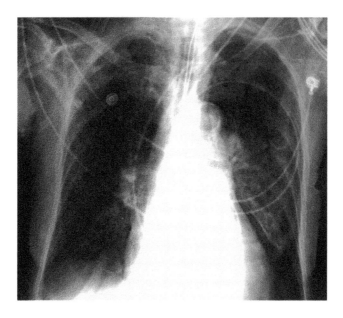

Discussion

The portable film reveals a patient who is markedly hyperaerated. This patient has chronic obstructive lung disease, and of course, you noticed what led to his symptoms. There is an absence of markings in the lower lung field; the characteristic deep sulcus sign indicates a moderate pneumothorax. The endotracheal tube is in good position.

CASE 17

This 19-year-old woman was brought to the emergency department comatose after an overdose. She had marked difficulty breathing and some degree of airway spasms. An attempt was made to intubate her. Marked difficulty was encountered and a film obtained.

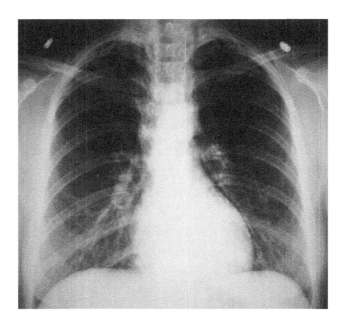

Discussion

Although no tubes or lines can be visualized in this film, it is interesting to note the extensive amount of air in this patient's mediastinum and neck and extending down alongside the cardiac shadow. Obviously, because of a very traumatic attempt at intubation, there was extravasation of air into the tissue surrounding the trachea, which then dissected down into the mediastinum. After this film, the patient was successfully intubated and then made a successful recovery. The patient's clinical symptomatology may precede radiographic findings, and initially, radiographic findings may be minimal to normal.

CASE 18

This patient with long-standing chronic lung disease came to the emergency department with respiratory insufficiency. An attempt was made to intubate him.

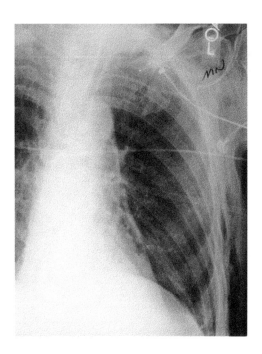

Discussion

The portable film reveals an endotracheal tube in good position. However, did you notice the subcutaneous emphysema on the left? A subtle finding is air present in the mediastinum and then tracking to the left chest wall. Would you do any other film?

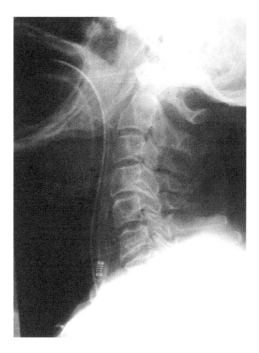

A lateral neck film reveals air dissecting in the soft tissues of the prevertebral space, which then dissected into the mediastinum and then out to the chest wall. A difficult intubation can lead to mediastinal air with subsequent air in soft tissues.

PNEUMONIA

CASE 19

This patient is 1 week postop for a Whipple procedure for carcinoma of the pancreas. He had been intubated for a week and began to spike temperatures.

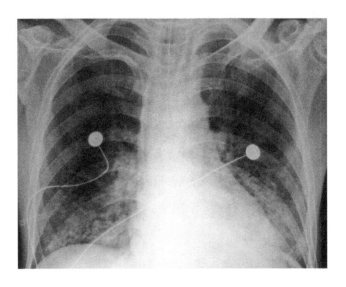

ICU Chest Radiology: Principles and Case Studies, by Harold Moskowitz
Copyright © 2010 John Wiley & Sons, Inc.

Discussion

The portable film reveals infiltrates bilaterally. Note the basilar position of the infiltrates, quite characteristic of a patient who has been intubated for a long period of time and who has developed the classic appearance of aspiration pneumonia, specifically a nosocomial infection after prolonged intubation. The area of infection depends on the position of the patient. Classically, the pneumonia is in the basilar segments and in the most posterior segments of the lung.

CASE 20

A patient with chronic obstructive lung disease came to the emergency department with an elevated temperature. A portable film was obtained on admission to the ICU.

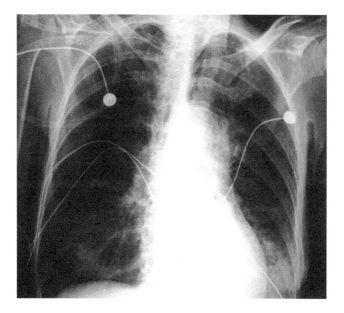

Discussion

Note that this film is somewhat hyperaerated, but still one cannot see through the heart to visualize the vascularity of the lower lobes.

In addition, one can see an area of infiltrate lateral to the left heart border, partially obliterating a portion of the left hemidiaphragm. The findings are all consistent with pneumonia in the left lower lobe.

CASE 21

A patient who was in a brawl and was stabbed in the abdomen and chest was admitted several days earlier with a pneumothrax and perforated bowel. On postop day 6, he developed spiking temperatures and marked shortness of breath.

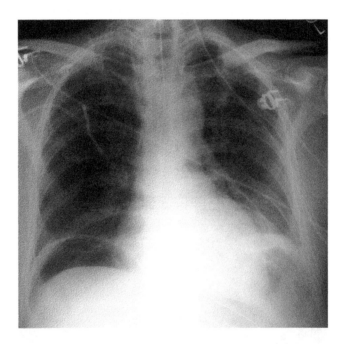

Discussion

There is a significant amount of intra-abdominal air postoperatively, and a Heimlich tube with the pigtail opened up in the right chest.

Of interest, of course, is the left lower lobe. There is elevation in the left hemidiaphragm, with obliteration of the most medial portion of it. There is consolidation of the medial basal segments of the left lower lobe as well as areas of mediastinal emphysema.

CASE 22

This 88-year-old patient with high fever was admitted from a nursing home.

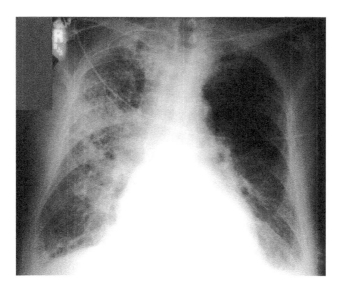

Discussion

On admission to the ICU, this patient's film revealed an extensive pneumonia in the right upper lobe and in the left lower lobe. Note the classic appearance of air alveolograms in the right upper lobe.

CASE 23

This patient has carcinoma of the colon, and a Dobhoff tube was placed in the stomach. This film is repeated from the text because several findings should be amplified.

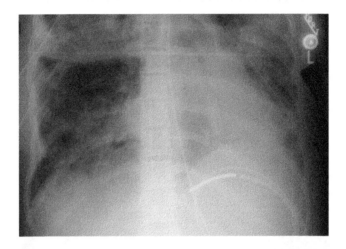

Discussion

Note the Dobhoff tube, which is coiled in the stomach. A feeding tube should be near or through the pylorus. Here, it is at the esophageal gastric junction. Does aspiration play a role in this patient's extensive bilateral pneumonias? Note the upper lobe is consolidated, with the fissure bulging downward secondary to gram negative organisms. There is also extensive infiltrate in the left lower lobr, with extensive air bronchograms and obliteration of the left hemidiaphragm. On the right side, there is a pneumonia obliterating the right cardiac border, indicating extensive pneumonia in the right middle lobe. In addition, a portion of the right hemidiaphragm is silhouetted, indicating a right basilar pneumonia.

CASE 24

This nursing home patient was admitted in the middle of the night with marked shortness of breath and a low-grade temperature. A portable film was obtained.

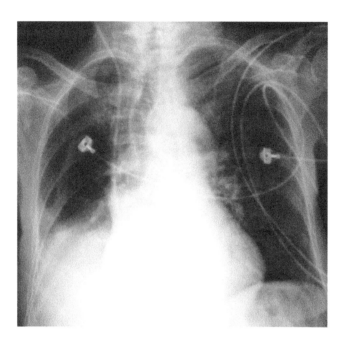

Discussion

On review of the film, the resident wanted to do a thoracentesis to remove the fluid in the right lower pleural space. You, of course, recognize that this is not fluid but rather consolidation in the right lower lobe. You can be sure of your finding since there is obliteration in the right hemidiaphragm, but the right cardiac border is easily seen. If there were fluid in the pleural space producing the density seen in the right lower lung field, it would obliterate the right cardiac border as well. Visualizing the right cardiac border indicates the right middle lobe is aerating. You correctly refuse to do a thoracentesis because the last thing the patient needs is pneumothrax, and you treat the patient with antibiotics for his consolidative pneumonia.

CASE 25

This 48-year-old woman with carcinoma of the breast treated with chemotherapy came to the ER with high fever and a white cell count of 800. She was admitted to the ICU, and a portable film was obtained.

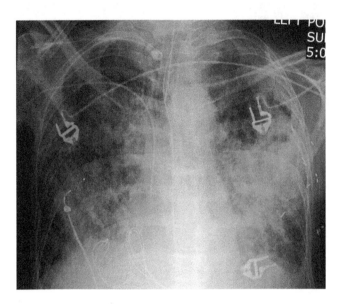

Discussion

The portable film reveals extensive bilateral pneumonia. There is a confluent area in middle left lung field as well as extensive pneumonia throughout the right lung with air alveolograms. The central line is seen in good position, as is an ET tube. The NG tube is just into the stomach, with the side hole in the esophagus. This should be advanced for fear of aspiration pneumonia.

CASE 26

This 43-year-old patient entered the emergency department with cough and fever. A portable film was obtained, and the patient was sent to the ICU.

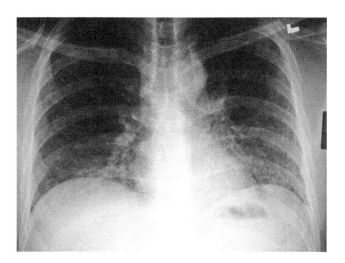

Discussion

The heart is normal. Did you notice the interstitial changes throughout both lung fields were somewhat more marked in the lower lung fields? This patient has full-blown AIDS, and this is a characteristic appearance of *Pneumocystis carinii* pneumonia.

CASE 27

This patient was sent to the ICU from the floor with an increased shortness of breath and high fever. A portable film was obtained.

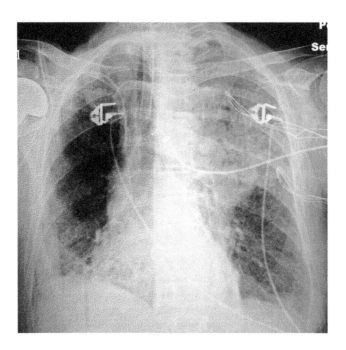

Discussion

Of course, you see the extensive infiltrate in the left upper lung field. Air bronchograms are seen throughout with a question of early cavitation. The entotracheal tube is in good position and the central line is in the upper part of the superior vena cava. The findings suggest extensive pneumonia with beginning cavitation, probably secondary to a staphylococcal pneumonia.

NODULAR PNEUMONIA

CASE 28

This is a portable film of a very sick patient who presented to the ER with shaking chills and fever. After the insertion of both an endotracheal tube and a chest tube, a portable film was taken.

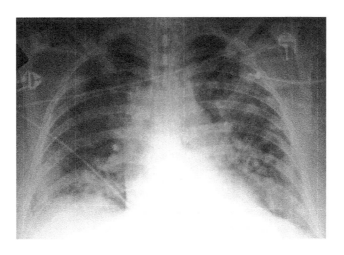

ICU Chest Radiology: Principles and Case Studies, by Harold Moskowitz
Copyright © 2010 John Wiley & Sons, Inc.

Discussion

Film reveals nodular masses throughout both lung fields. These nodular masses are bilateral, with indistinct borders. Occasionally, one may see a small area of breakdown.

What would be your differential diagnosis? Of course metastatic disease must be considered. Then, one should always consider granulomatous disease, with fairly extensive involvement. Another often overlooked diagnosis is septic emboli. The fuzziness and lack of definition, and what may be an occasional area of necrosis, suggests the diagnosis of septic emboli. Is the patient an IV drug abuser? Listen to the heart in the region of the tricuspid valve, looking for insufficiency, and then order an echocardiogram to perhaps demonstrate material on the tricuspid valve indicating endocarditis. When interviewed, the patient admitted that he had been an intravenous drug user for a short period of time months earlier.

PULMONARY EDEMA

CASE 29

This patient was admitted to the hospital with marked shortness of breath after suffering a large posterior lateral wall infarct.

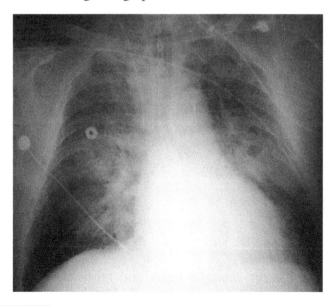

ICU Chest Radiology: Principles and Case Studies, by Harold Moskowitz
Copyright © 2010 John Wiley & Sons, Inc.

Discussion

Portable film reveals the heart to be at the upper limits of normal. Note the classic appearance of pulmonary edema with bilateral perihilar fluid, loss of definition of the pulmonary vascularity, and a fairly classic bat wing appearance. The patient has had an intraortic pump balloon inserted, which is in good position. A central line and endotracheal tube are also in good position.

CASE 30

This patient, who has severe coronary artery disease and congestive myopathy, was admitted to the ICU.

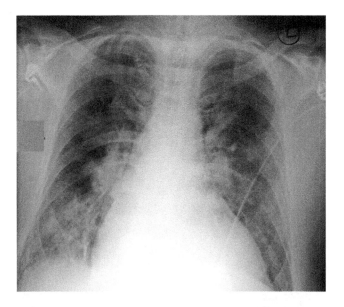

Discussion

This patient has an enlarged heart and fairly classic findings of increased flow to the upper lobe, so-called cephalization, as well as perivascular cuffing.

CASE 31

This patient entered the emergency department with dyspnea.

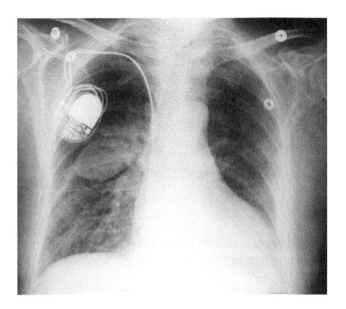

Discussion

The patient has a bipolar pacer. What is interesting is the density in the right middle lung field. This elliptical density represents fluid trapped the oblique fissure. Normally fluid is free in the pleural space, but here fluid accumulates between the two layers of the pleura and is "pinched" off in two areas due to fibrosis and scarring, so a pool of fluid develops in this area, producing this characteristic appearance. This may disappear spontaneously and rapidly, and this density is sometimes referred to as a vanishing tumor.

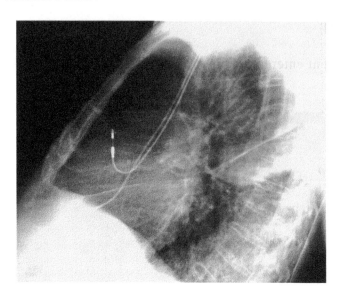

Discussion

The lateral film reveals to better advantage the position of the loculated fluid posteriorly in the major fissure.

CASE 32

This patient had revascularization surgery for the second time and is having increasing dyspnea.

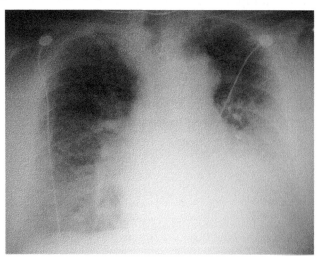

Discussion

The portable film reveals some degree of vascular congestion but note the characteristic Kerley lines in the periphery of the lung.

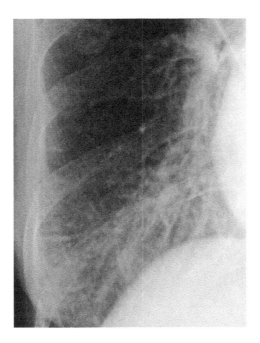

A close-up view reveals the characteristic appearance of interstitial fluid and fluid in the lymphatics adjacent to the pleura. Note the pleural stripe laterally, which represents subvisceral pleural fluid. Fluid in the interstium of the lung is being carried by the lymphatics back toward the pleural surface, and the fluid accumulates underneath the visceral pleura, producing this lateral stripe.

CASE 33

The patient presented to the emergency department with classic congestive failure.

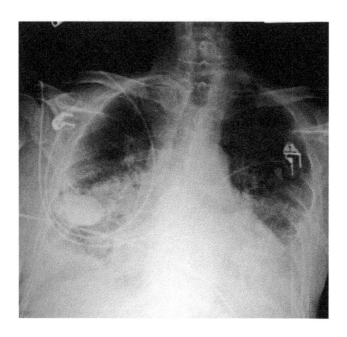

Discussion

The film reveals cardiomegaly and an elevated left main stem bronchus, indicating this patient has left atrial enlargement. There is straightening the left cardiac border as well as left ventricular enlargement. The findings suggest the diagnosis of mitral insufficiency.

Of interest is the classic appearance of loculated fluid in the horizontal fissure. After fluid treatment, these densities often go away.

CASE 34

This 39-year-old patient entered the emergency department with marked shortness of breath. A portable film was obtained.

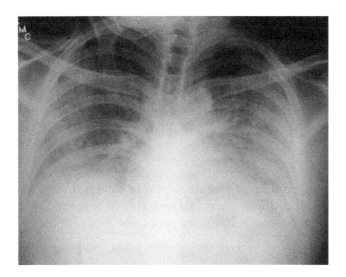

Discussion

This patient has small lung volumes with pulmonary edema. There is an area of atelectasis in the left upper lung field. This patient had been snorting cocaine and came in with an acute MI and congestive failure.

ARDS

CASE 35

This 58-year-old patient sustained severe bilateral leg trauma in an auto accident and had been in the ICU for several days when he developed increasing respiratory problems.

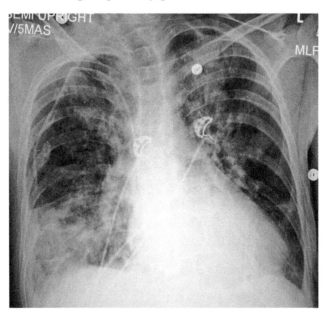

Discussion

This patient's film reveals an extensive confluent infiltrate in the right lower lung field. One could assume that this represents an extensive pneumonia. There are however, are other patchy infiltrates, including one in the left upper lobe and probably an infiltrate of the left lower lobe, posteriorly, behind the heart. Note that there are air bronchograms in the right lower lobe. The patient was not running a fever, and his white count was within normal limits. The findings most likely represent ARDS.

CASE 36

This 32-year-old patient had a cholycystectomy, subsequently developed a bile leak, and had to go back to the OR. Progressive respiratory problems ensued, and this film was obtained 5 days later.

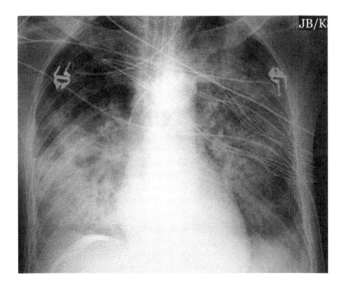

Discussion

The film reveals extensive confluent bilateral infiltrates. Do not mistake this for failure. The heart is normal, and the infiltrates are not perihilar. They are more extensive in the right lower lobe, with several patchy areas in the right upper lobe, and extensive alveolar changes on the left. Previously, the patient had several small areas of infiltrate, but now there is coalescence and extension. This is all due to an alveolar leak and extensive ARDS. A left-sided central line, placed via the internal jugular route, is seen. The endotracheal tube is in fairly good position, but probably slightly higher than one would like to see.

CASE 37

This 62-year-old patient with pancreatitis was admitted to the hospital and developed severe respiratory difficulty after 7 days.

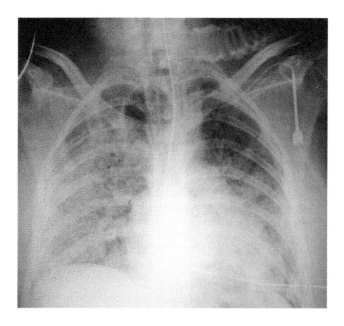

Discussion

The film reveals almost total opacification and coalescence of infiltrate in the right lung. A large air space, probably pneumatocele, can be seen in the right upper lobe. Extensive coalescence can be seen on the left, and there are air bronchograms bilaterally. There is some mediastinal emphysema, indicating that the patient, due to the difficulty in ventilating these lungs, has developed barotrauma with mediastinal air.

CASE 38

A patient with extensive bilateral infiltrates was sent for CT because of the possibility, seen on the plain film, of mediastinal emphysema.

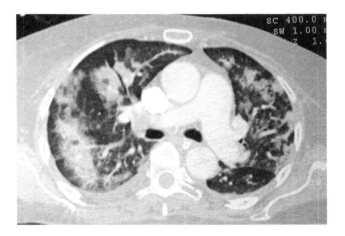

Discussion

CT of the chest reveals an extensive patchy area of alveolar density, bilaterally. There is no evidence of mediastinal emphysema. The CT reveals the coalescence of these alveolar densities, secondary to increased permeability of the membrane associated with type II pneumocyte damage. This infiltrate consists of a PAS positively stained material, much like the material in hyaline membrane disease in the neonate.

CASE 39

A 42-year-old patient with progressive respiratory insufficiency has been in the ICU for 5 days.

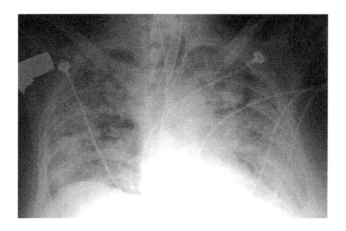

Discussion

The portable film reveals prominent extensive bilateral alveolar densities. There is consolidation in the left lower lobe. Note the endotracheal tube, which is in good position. The cuff surrounding the tube is inflated beyond the walls of the trachea. This is due to a persistent air leak and the stiff lungs this patient developed secondary to the extensive infiltrate throughout most of the alveolar cells. Care must be taken not to overdistend the trachea and not to permit the balloon to remain totally expanded for a prolonged period of time. Ischemia and necrosis can be the result.

CASE 40

A 72-year-old patient went to the hospital through the emergency department after having sustained severe pelvic trauma in a car accident 6 days earlier.

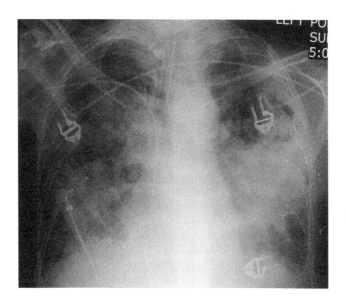

Discussion

Note the extensive opacification of almost the entire left lung and a good portion of the right lung, including the right middle lobe and probably part of the upper lobe. There is some aeration in both these areas. Although a good portion of this may well be due to ARDS, the possibility of co-existing pneumonia must be always entertained. Recognizing this and beginning antibiotics earlier will permit the patient to heal that much faster.

CASE 41

This patient presented after hip surgery with considerable shortness of breath.

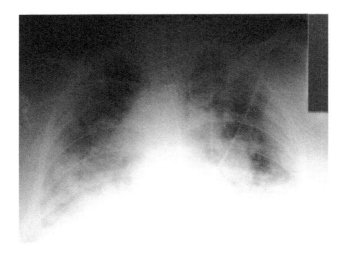

Discussion

Initially, the patient developed area of atelectasis and then several areas of confluent density, probably pneumonia. This film, taken 10 days later, reveals extensive areas of alveolar density, probably representing both pneumonia and ARDS.

PULMONARY EMBOLUS

CASE 42

This 41-year-old male came to the ER with chest pain and shortness of breath. He had been on a long plane trip 3 days earlier, and noted swelling of his left leg the day before coming to the ER.

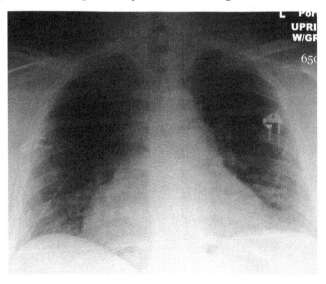

ICU Chest Radiology: Principles and Case Studies, by Harold Moskowitz
Copyright © 2010 John Wiley & Sons, Inc.

Discussion

The portable film reveals prominent right side of the heart. What would you do now?

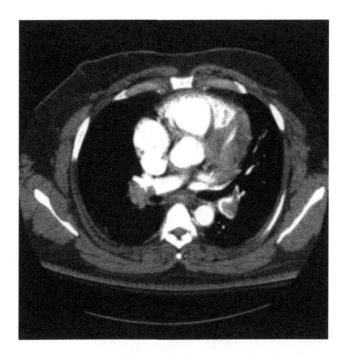

In a patient with a swollen leg, chest pain, and especially with a large right-sided heart, the diagnosis of pulmonary embolus must be considered. The standard of care today should be a CT angiogram. The CT angiogram reveals extensive pulmonary emboli in both the right and left arteries.

ATELECTASIS AND COLLAPSE

CASE 43

This patient came to the ICU several days earlier with a left lower lobe pneumonia. He has had progressive respiratory difficulties and was intubated 3 days earlier. A repeat film was just taken.

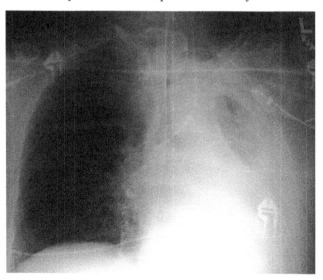

ICU Chest Radiology: Principles and Case Studies, by Harold Moskowitz
Copyright © 2010 John Wiley & Sons, Inc.

Discussion

The portable film reveals almost total opacification of the left lung, with loss of the left hemidiaphragm and the left cardiac border. Only a small bit of aerating lung is seen in the central portion of the lung. There is a mild shift of the mediastinum to the left, indicating loss of volume. We can see the obstruction of the left main bronchus, with a cutoff sign. This patient had a large mucus plug, causing collapse.

Did you notice the position of the left internal jugular central line? Note its low descent and crossing over to the right, indicating a persistent left superior vena cava, with the vessel rejoining the superior vena cava just above the region of the right atrium.

CASE 44

This patient came to the emergency department with dyspnea and shortness of breath. A portable film raised questions.

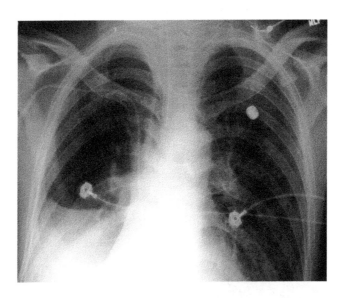

Discussion

The portable film reveals a density in the right lower lung field. Note that the cardiac border is easily seen, and the horizontal fissure is somewhat depressed. The right diaphragmatic border is not seen, indicating this is a large consolidation of the right lower lobe. The differential diagnosis is between atelectasis and pneumonia of the right lower lobe. The question of fluid can be completely eliminated by the visualization of the right cardiac border.

CASE 45

A newborn developed marked shortness of breath and a portable film was obtained.

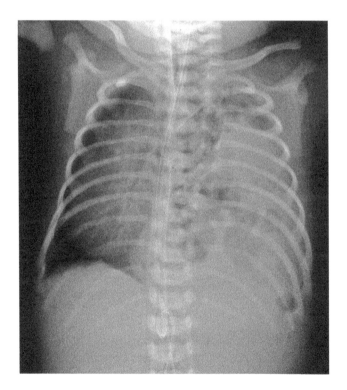

Discussion

The portable film establishes the diagnosis in this newborn. Note that there is no gas in the abdomen. The left hemithorax has a peculiar configuration, with both gas- and solid-contained structures. There is some shift of the mediastinum to the right. The findings are all characteristic of the absence of the left hemidiaphragm, with herniation of the GI tract into the left lung. This is almost always associated with hypoplasia of the left pulmonary artery.

CASE 46

This 54-year-old alcoholic was found unconscious late one Saturday night and brought to the emergency department.

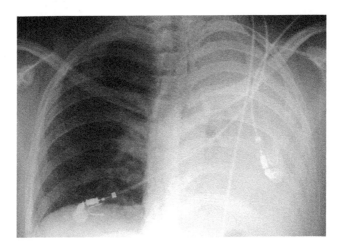

Discussion

The portable film reveals total opacification of the left hemithorax. What do you think is the etiology of this opacification? Can this be fluid? Clearly there is shift of the mediastinum to the left, indicating that there is loss of volume in the left lung. It cannot be fluid because the left chest is opacified; if this were fluid there would be a shift of the mediastinum to the right. The patient had aspirated while lying on his left side, with a piece of food stuck in his left mainstem bronchus, causing collapse of the left lung.

CASE 47

This patient came in with marked shortness of breath, and dyspnea.

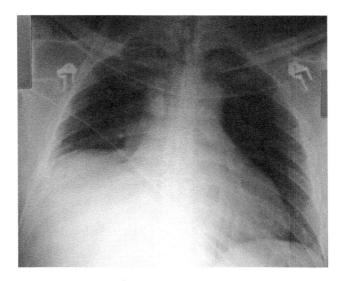

Discussion

A portable film reveals a density in the right lower lung. There is obliteration of the right hemidiaphragm as well as of the right cardiac border. What is the etiology of this density? One must consider whether there is an effusion present. There is no evidence of a meniscus, and what one sees is lung reaching to the horizontal fissure. The most likely diagnosis is opacification of the right middle and right lower lobes. To be certain, one could do an ultrasound to see if there is fluid present. However, the configuration of the horizontal fissure certainly makes one suspect that this configuration is of collapse and opacification of the right, lower, and middle lobes. Clinical evaluation is important for understanding the etiology. If the patient is running a temperature and has an elevated white count, this most likely represents lobar pneumonia, although atelectasis of the right lower and right middle lobe is certainly a diagnostic possibility. Actually, this patient had a tumor in the bronchus intermedius, causing obstruction and collapse.

CASE 48

This 73-year-old woman presented one evening to the emergency department with severe anterior chest pain. The portable film was obtained.

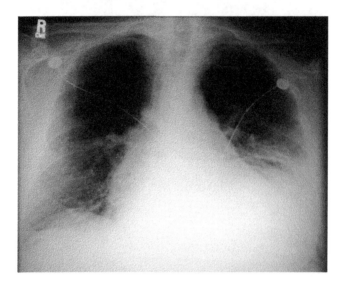

Discussion

This film was interpreted by the emergency department physician to show an elevated left hemidiaphragm with cardiomegaly. The patient was thought to have angina, and she was taken to the catheterization laboratory, where coronary angiography found only minor coronary artery disease. Do you have an alternative diagnosis?

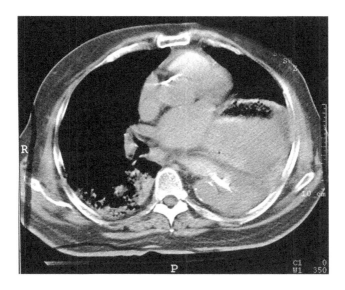

When the film was reviewed in the morning with the radiologist, the possibility of an alternative diagnosis was raised. The radiologist suggested that this configuration represented a large hiatal hernia. Because of the severe pain, the possibility that this patient had a volvus was considered. CT study revealed a good portion of the stomach in the chest.

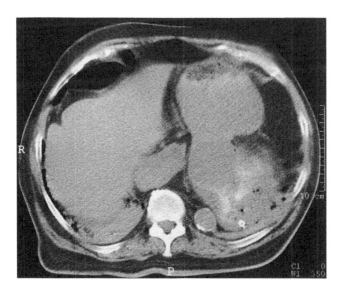

The patient drank a small amount of contrast, but the fundus of the stomach reveals air and a peculiar configuration. The patient went to the operating room, which revealed that an organo-axial rotation and volvulus of the stomach had occurred, with necrosis of the stomach. She underwent resection of the stomach but died several hours later.

CASE 49

This patient was admitted to the ICU for dyspnea and shortness of breath. He was intubated and film was obtained.

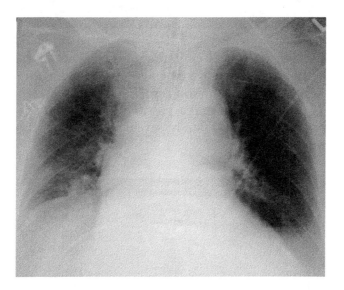

Discussion

Note the position of the endotracheal tube, which is just at the carina and probably just into the right mainstem bronchus. In spite of this, notice that the right hemidiaphragm is elevated and there is loss of volume in the right lower lobe. The right cardiac border is visualized. The findings are secondary to atelectasis and partial collapse of the right lower lobe.

CASE 50

This film is of a newborn who was intubated due to respiratory distress.

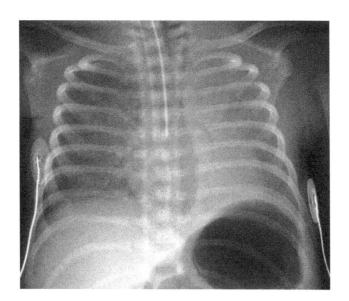

Discussion

You notice that the entotracheal tube is into the right mainstem bronchus. Note that the left hemidiaphragm is elevated and there is lack of aeration in the left lung. The endotracheal tube in the right mainstem bronchus is partially occluding the left mainstem bronchus, causing loss of volume and some degree of atelectasis of the left lung.

CASE 51

This patient was admitted with shortness of breath and a diagnosis of atelectasis of the left lung from an outside hospital to the ICU.

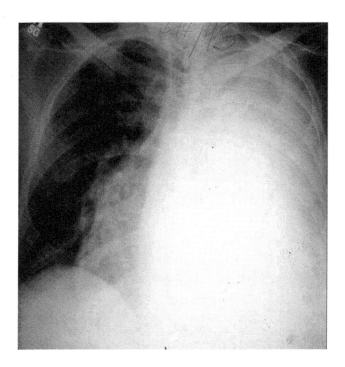

Discussion

Portable film reveals total opacification of the left hemithorax. The initial diagnosis was atelectasis and collapse of the left lung. You, of course, can see that this is not true. Note the position of the mediastinum and the trachea. The trachea and mediastinum are shifted to the right, indicating that instead of loss of volume, there is a density that is moving the mediastinum to the right. While a large tumor could produce this, most likely there is a huge, left-sided effusion, with a shift of the mediastinum to the right, and not atelectasis of the left lung.

INDEX

Abscess, 92
Absorption
  coefficient, 7
  of scatter, 9
Acute lung injury (ALI), 79–81, 83
Acute myocardial infarction, 73, 76,
    151. *See also* Myocardial
    infarction
Acute respiratory distress
    syndrome (ARDS)
  case studies, 152–158
  characteristics of, 50, 60, 70,
    78–79
  co-existing pneumonia, 157–158
  CT scans, 83–84
  defined, 80
  diagnosis, 80–81
  etiologies, 80, 82–83
  exudate phase of, 81–82

first radiographic abnormalities,
    81
infiltrates, 153–154
mortality rates, 81
radiographic appearance of,
    81–83
recovery phase, 85
severe, 83
Adenopathy, 18
Adhesive atelectasis, 90
AIDS patients, 65, 141
Air alveolograms, 137, 140
Air bronchograms, 18, 60–61,
    63–64, 79, 82–85, 90–93, 138,
    142, 153–154
Air cysts, 55
Air-fluid levels, 44
Air space density, 78
Air to tissue ratio, 47

ICU Chest Radiology: Principles and Case Studies, by Harold Moskowitz
Copyright © 2010 John Wiley & Sons, Inc.

Printed and bound by CPI Group (UK) Ltd, Croydon, CR0 4YY

16/04/2025

14658523-0001